Improving Speech and Eating Skills in Children with Autism Spectrum Disorders

An Oral-Motor Program for Home and School

Maureen A. Flanagan, MA, CCC-SLP

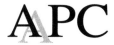

©2008 Autism Asperger Publishing Company
P. O. Box 23173
Shawnee Mission, Kansas 66283-0173
877-277-8254 • www.asperger.net

Publisher's Cataloging-in-Publication

Flanagan, Maureen A.
    Improving speech and eating skills in children with autism spectrum
    disorders : an oral-motor program for home and school / Maureen A.
    Flanagan. – 1st ed. – Shawnee Mission, Kan. : Autism Asperger
    Pub. Co., c2008.

        p. ; cm.
        ISBN: 978-1-934575-23-9
        LCCN: 2008924314
        Includes bibliographical references.

        1. Autistic children--Language. 2. Mastication disorders.
    3. Psychomotor disorders in children. 4. Speech therapy for
    children. 5. Autistic children--Treatment. I. Title.

RJ506.A9 F53   2008 2008924314
618.92/85882–dc22   0804

This book is designed in Minion.

Printed in the United States of America.

This book is dedicated to my husband, Jack, and my daughters, Meghan, Emma, and Julia, for their continued support and encouragement.

Special thanks to the children and their parents, my father, Andrew Flanagan, my brother, Christopher Flanagan, and my colleagues Kathy Rodriguez, Donna Surber, Susan Zwany, Vicki Mechner, and Dr. Janet Powell.

– M. A. Flanagan

Table of Contents

)X(

Introduction

Suzie, age 5, has a diagnosis of autism spectrum disorder. She has a limited diet, preferring crunchy foods, such as pretzels, that are quick and easy to chew. Suzie rejects slimy foods, such as canned peaches, meats, foods with lumps, and most fruits and vegetables. She is a very messy eater and often stuffs her mouth with food. Her parents dread brushing her teeth because of the way she fights them. She sometimes gags when they approach with her toothbrush. Suzie spontaneously produces some single words and phrases but does not consistently imitate words and phrases after her parents and teachers. She produces a limited variety of speech sounds.

Suzie will continue to have difficulty imitating words and phrases, expanding the variety of speech sounds, accepting new foods, and tolerating tactile input from others until this aversion to tactile input is addressed through oral-motor treatment.

Evaluation of oral-motor skills has often been overlooked in treatment programs for children with autism spectrum disorders (ASD), partly due to a general lack of considering the development of the whole child. Thus, programs have often encouraged verbal imitation without focusing on the child's ability to process the sensory information and then produce the components of movements needed to produce a sound or a syllable. In the case of Suzie, this child is hypersensitive to tactile input inside the mouth. Suzie does not want to move the tongue vertically to the top of the mouth to produce a /d/ or an /n/ sound because it does not feel good to make contact with the palate or roof of the mouth. In fact, as we saw in the vignette, she may even gag when her tongue makes contact there.

Oral-motor development is part of normal development and must be considered when looking at the child and her treatment program. They are the components that form the foundation of the sensory motor patterns that are practiced during the development of the simple as well as complex skills used while eating and speaking.

Children with ASD, to varying degrees, are unable to register and modulate sensory information in one or more of the sensory systems (Ayers, 1979; Henry & Myles, 2007; Yack, Aquilla, & Sutton, 2002). This interferes with the ability to initiate movements, to plan movements, to sequence movements, and to develop a feedback system. All of these inhibit the development of oral-motor skills, in turn affecting eating, speech production, and communication.

Brief Overview of Sensory Processing and Oral-Motor Skills

Ayers, in her book *Sensory Integration and the Child* (1979), documents the symptoms of poor sensory processing that can affect oral-motor development in children with ASD. The number of sensory systems that are not registering and modulating information affects the level of severity of the child's dysfunction.

For example, the child who is able to process information through her proprioceptive, tactile, and visual systems but not through the auditory system will present a different level of functioning from the child who is not processing information well from any of these systems.

The first child would have a sense of where his body is in space, accept being approached by others, and possibly gain information by reading. But he would be unable to follow verbal directions, need frequent repetition of verbal language, and possibly be using scripted language to communicate. The second child would easily become overstimulated by information, causing him to over-react or under-react and become defensive. This child would present with a more severe level of dysfunction, given his oral-motor, eating, and speech production.

Children with Differing Needs

Ayers (1979) cites three areas where children with autism have poor sensory processing – registering sensory information, modulating sensory input, and initiating movement. Each area is briefly described in the following.

Registering Sensory Information

Thomas, 7 years old, was attending to a siren from a fire engine in the distance and not to his teacher leading a lesson. A hand on his shoulder from his teacher assistant and the use of a microphone by the teacher to amplify her voice brought his attention back to the lesson.

Children with ASD often do not pay attention to information that is important, such as speech sounds. For example, instead of attending to speech, the child may attend to a background noise, such as the humming of a fan, not noticed by others around her. According to Ayers (1979), in such cases, the part of the brain that "decides" which information to attend to and what to do about that information is not "registering well."

Emily, a 5-year-old girl with a diagnosis of ASD, had difficulty registering touch sensations. She never felt drool on her chin or food on her face. Emily also stuffed food in her mouth with no awareness that her mouth was already full. Emily's mother wondered why she had to constantly tell her daughter to wipe her face or take small bites and swallow.

This is commonly seen in children with ASD, but in varying degrees. Indeed, the ability to take in and respond to information is inconsistent within and across individuals. Motivation, strong sensations, and firm input are needed in order for these children to respond optimally to sensory input.

Modulating Sensory Input

Terry, an 8-year-old boy with a diagnosis of ASD, had difficulty modulating touch input. He could not tolerate the way his clothes felt against his skin. He spent a lot of his time pulling and tugging at his clothes. He frequently stood up and pulled his pants up at the waist. Instead of filtering out this touch sensation, all he could think about was how his clothes felt at that moment. This made it difficult to attend to another child trying to talk with him or to his teacher during a lesson (Yack et al., 2002).

The brains of many children with ASD are unable to control sensory input, causing them to receive too much input or not enough. In other words, the child is unable to balance the sensory input (Henry & Myles, 2007). In the first situation, the child is bombarded by input from one or more sensory systems. In the second, the child is not getting enough stimulation and, therefore, may crave input from one or more sensory systems.

Another example involving the tactile system (touch) is the child who needs strong, firm touch in order to register input but then quickly becomes overloaded and reacts defensively. This child is unable to regulate and integrate this input into his body awareness and make sense of the input once it is registered. This can result in oral-motor planning problems. An example is the child who has difficulty moving her mouth when requested to do so. She cannot stick out her tongue when asked or when given a visual model. However, the child can be seen to stick out her tongue while automatically licking a lollipop. It is difficult to plan movements when you do not have a good sense of your body. Further, when the child cannot organize and plan simple movements, he has trouble developing more complex behaviors such as speech production. In brief, the ability to plan movements depends, in part, on the accuracy of the child's touch system.

Initiating Movement

Jason, a 6-year-old boy with a diagnosis of ASD, had difficulty initiating movement. He would respond to an adult or a child who greeted him with a "good morning" or "hi" by saying the same word(s) or phrase(s) back. Jason would also repeat the phrase with his own name, if that was initially said to him. However, he would never initiate a greeting to anyone. His parents could not understand this since he could say the words so clearly in response to others.

According to Ayers (1979), the third area of sensory processing that can present challenges to a child with ASD is the ability and the motivation to initiate movements.

Actions need to be known or meaningful to the child before she engages in them on her own. That is, the child may have the motor ability to perform an action, but not until the movement is practiced repeatedly will it become meaningful so that she can initiate it. For example, some children with ASD have difficulty initiating communication even though they have a vocabulary of 50 or more words. "Initiation is more challenging than responding because children have to create their own independent thoughts and ideas and are not able to get ideas from or build on someone else's questions or comments" (Henry & Myles, 2007, p. 76).

Why This Book?

As illustrated, for children with sensory processing difficulties, sensory input must be presented in such a way that the child can register, regulate, integrate, and organize it – and consequently respond. The oral-motor program presented in this book describes an environment where sensory information is presented in this manner so the child can accept and use oral input and activities to improve oral-motor function during eating, speech production, and nonverbal and verbal communication. Because the program is presented in the same way and the same order each time, the child comes to know what to expect and, therefore, finds it easier to process the information that is presented. This is particularly important for children on the autism spectrum, who tend to crave routines and sameness.

In my professional work, I have met many families with children as young as 3 and as old as 15 years of age who have never worked inside their child's mouth or had a professional work inside their child's mouth. The histories are all very typical.

- The child has a limited diet.
- The child gags easily.
- The child does not like to have his or her teeth brushed.
- The child produces a limited number of speech sounds.
- The child does not consistently imitate or initiate words or phrases.

Working on oral-motor skills will help to expand the child's diet, accept oral input from a toothbrush and the oral structures, increase the number of sounds that are produced, and assist with imitation and initiation of speech production. Our goal is to improve critical skills that are part of daily basic routine and form the foundation for higher-level functioning.

This book gives parents and teachers knowledge, techniques, and activities to enable them to work on these oral-motor skills with the children in their lives. It also gives parents and teachers the reason, or "the why," for working on these skills. This author has worked with many families who have said, "We used to use a chew tube and Nuk™ brush. I don't know where those are any more." Sadly, these families had stopped using these tools because no one had explained to them why it is important to continue working on oral awareness, oral stability, oral strength, and oral sensitivity.

Specifically, this book will show how oral-motor treatment helps to increase oral awareness, normalize oral sensitivity, improve oral strength and stability, facilitate more typical movement patterns, increase separation and grading of movement, and improve the child's overall ability to initiate movements. This means that with oral-motor treatment, the child will become aware of how the lips, tongue, and cheeks are moving and will become able to purposefully move these structures for eating, speech production, or sequenced language. There will be separation of movement with stability so he can move the tongue, lips, and cheeks independently from the lower jaw. These movement patterns influence the child's ability to eat, drink, speak, communicate verbally and non-verbally, control drooling, and gain information from the environment. They also affect the child's ability to produce survival responses such as coughing, swallowing, and gagging. Although the information written here is meant for children with a diagnosis of ASD, it can be used with any child who is exhibiting delayed or disordered oral-motor patterns.

Benefits of Oral-Motor Treatment
1. **Increased oral awareness:** The child develops an image of the oral structures and is able to use them for purposeful movements.
2. **Improved oral sensitivity:** The child is able to react discriminately rather than defensively to tactile input to and with the oral structures.
3. **Improved muscle strength:** This gives us our ability to move against gravity and maintain our position in space. It assists with giving stability to the oral structures.
4. **Improved separation and grading of oral movements:** This enables the child to produce the precise, independent movements needed for eating and speech production.
5. **More typical movement patterns:** Oral-motor treatment reduces the need for compensatory movement patterns and encourages the use of more typical movement patterns to develop.
6. **Improved ability to initiate movement:** If the child has a better sense of the oral structures, it becomes easier to produce volitional movement.

Overview of the Book

In Chapter 1, terms often associated with ASD are defined with examples of behaviors associated with them. Chapter 2 describes the evaluation process so that parents and teachers know what to expect from the therapist performing an oral-motor evaluation. This chapter also includes an explanation of normal, delayed, and abnormal oral-motor development. A table overviewing typical oral-motor, eating, and speech development from birth through age 3 is found here.

Chapter 3 defines the environment needed for a successful treatment session. This environment is structured so that optimum processing of information and movements is elicited from the child. An oral-motor program as well as the materials required for an oral-motor kit are included, along with suggested activities. Foods that enhance and inhibit mature movement patterns are also listed. Chapter 4 gives examples of how to include the oral-motor program into the child's daily routines at home and in the classroom, along with ideas for promoting mature movement patterns throughout the day. Also found in Chapter 4 are case stories that describe boys, with a diagnosis of autism, who prospered from using the oral-motor program. Chapter 5 presents complementary therapies that have been used to promote mature movement patterns in children with a variety of movement and processing disorders with an emphasis on how they can benefit a child with ASD. Finally, the Appendix contains (a) the Oral-Motor/Eating/Speech Checklist, (b) Material for Oral-Motor Kit, (c) Oral-Motor Data Sheets, (d) Glossary, and (e) Resources.

X

CHAPTER 1

Conditions Associated with Autism Spectrum Disorders

A utism is one of the five pervasive developmental disorders (PDDs) listed in the *Diagnostic and Statistical Manual of Mental disorders* (4th Edition, Text Revision: DSM-IV; American Psychiatric Association [APA, 2000]). Children with autism spectrum disorders (ASD) exhibit a broad range of behaviors and levels of severity. Briefly, these are defined as a severe deficit in social interactions, language, communication and play, with stereotypic, repetitive behaviors and a narrow range of interests (Rapin, 1997). The DSM-IV (as cited in Yack et al., 2002) describes children with autistic disorder as having poor social skills, impaired communication skills, and stereotypic behaviors. Specific communication characteristics include poor processing of speech sounds, an unusual vocal tone, and difficulty understanding, sequencing and using words. Although not specified as a characteristic of ASD in the DSM-IV, sensory issues also appear to be inherent in individuals with this exceptionality (Henry & Myles, 2007).

Thus, certain behaviors present in children with ASD are related to hyper- (over) or hypo- (under) reactions to sensory input. This makes it difficult to gain useful information from sensory experiences and pay attention, a prerequisite for learning. Therefore, intervention needs to help the child attain a state of calm and alertness, organize sensory information, and develop a feedback system so that learning can take place (King, 1991). The treatment environment and oral-motor program described in Chapter 3 are structured such that the child with ASD can become calm and alert, organize sensory information, develop a feedback system, process speech sounds, use sequenced words, and follow directions.

Humans need large amounts of sensory stimulation in order to organize simple inputs into complex information or perceptions. Most of this stimulation comes from the vestibular, proprioceptive, and tactile systems, and, to a lesser extent, the auditory system. It is not surprising, therefore, that many of the unique behaviors exhibited by children with ASD, such as spinning, rocking, pacing, and jumping, are related to these systems, which are major sources of input. Thus, these behaviors are the child's attempt to become more organized and calm (King, 1991).

The auditory, proprioceptive, vestibular, and tactile systems will be described in this chapter. It is important to understand how a problem with the child's ability to register, modulate, and respond to information from each of these sensory systems may affect how you approach, converse, and work with the child.

Also described in this chapter are conditions often associated with ASD such as muscle tone, dysarthria, and apraxia. This background information is necessary for understanding the reasons behind the treatment environment, as well as the language and treatment techniques used in the oral-motor treatment program presented in Chapter 3.

Functions of Selected Sensory Systems

We will start by looking at selected sensory systems (see Table 1.1).

Table 1.1 Location and Functions of the Sensory Systems		
System	**Location**	**Function**
Auditory (hearing)	Inner ear – stimulated by air/sound waves.	Provides information about sounds in the environment (loud, soft, high, low, near, far).
Proprioception (body awareness)	Muscles and joints – activated by muscle contractions and movement.	Provides information about where a certain body part is and how it is moving.
Vestibular (balance)	Inner ear – stimulated by head movements and input from other senses, especially visual.	Provides information about where our body is in space, and whether or not we or our surroundings are moving. Tells about speed and direction of movement.
Tactile (touch)	Skin – density of cell distribution varies throughout the body. Areas of greatest density include mouth, hands, and genitals.	Provides information about the environment and object qualities (touch, pressure, texture, hard, soft, sharp, dull, heat, cold, pain).

From: *Asperger Syndrome and Sensory Issues – Practical Solutions for Making Sense of the World* by B. S. Myles, K. T. Cook, N. E. Miller, L. Rinner, and L. A. Robbins, 2000, Shawnee Mission, KS: Autism Asperger Publishing Company. Used with permission.

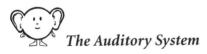 *The Auditory System*

"The ear is a sensory organ far more complex than other sensory organs" (Moller, 2006, p. 1). Our auditory system includes our ears and their complex central auditory pathways, ending in the cortex of the temporal lobes of the brain. The major parts of this system are the outer, middle, and inner ear and the central nervous system (Yost, 2002). The auditory system receives, encodes, transmits, and decodes sound signals that enable us to process instructions and information (Lawrence, 1971). It is here that sound is analyzed, primarily for frequency by filtering (Yost, 2002). As part of this process, unnecessary information is filtered out (Lawrence, 1971).

Children with ASD may hear all sounds at the same level and become overwhelmed by all the auditory information, making it difficult for them to attend to and follow what someone is saying to them. That is, they are unable to filter out unnecessary information and pay attention to what is most important in a given situation, such as speech production (Hoekman, 2005). They might be *hypersensitive* to certain sounds, causing them to cover their ears or make noises to block out the sound. When this happens, they are obviously unable to attend to any auditory input. Children may also close their eyes or put their head down on the table. You might even see them appear to be focusing on something in the distance to help deal with incoming stimuli.

Some children are *hyposensitive* to auditory information, causing them not to respond to input that others typically respond to. These children may stare blankly at the person talking with them until the message is repeated three, five, or more times. Gestures and sign language may need to be added in order to get a response. For example, the adult might point to the chair or produce the sign for "sit" before the child moves over to the chair and sits down.

It is important to understand that the same child can exhibit both of these types of behavior to different auditory information on the same day or be able to receive a certain amount of auditory information without difficulty one day but not the next. This is often confusing to parents, teachers, or caretakers. The difference in behavior is caused by the amount of sensory information the child has had to process over the course of that day; that is, we are often talking about a cumulative effect. This is why the amount of input provided during the oral-motor program is modified according the child's ability to process information at that moment.

Table 1.2 highlights some common difficulties in processing auditory stimuli and corresponding behavioral manifestations.

Table 1.2 Challenges Related to Processing Auditory Stimuli	
• Difficulty processing auditory stimuli	1. Becomes overwhelmed by auditory information 2. Does not pay attention to speech 3. Has difficulty following directions 4. Focuses on background noises
• Hypersensitive to auditory stimulation	1. Attempts to "block" auditory information by placing hands over ears or making sounds 2. Becomes upset or aggressive upon hearing certain sounds
• Hyposensitive to auditory stimulation	1. Needs repetition of auditory information 2. Needs "wait time" after receiving auditory information before responding

 The Proprioceptive System

The proprioceptive system gives us unconscious, automatic information from the sensory receptors in our muscles and joints about the position of our body and changes of position in space and movement (King, 2002b). For example, this system enables us to automatically guide our movements and adjust our position in space so we don't fall out of a chair or are able to move down off of a step (Hoekman, 2005). A sound proprioceptive system allows us to focus on what we want to do rather than on how we are going to do it because we have an awareness of our body in space. Further, the input from the proprioceptive system is calming and enables us to feel safe in our bodies.

Children with ASD often do not get the right amount of input from their proprioceptive system. As a result, they do not always know what their body is doing or how to make it do what they want it to do. An example would be the child who has difficulty walking down the hall at school and needs to be constantly touching the wall to orient himself. Poor processing of information from the proprioceptive system makes it difficult to produce coordinated movements and contributes to problems with motor planning – "the ability to plan and carry out an unfamiliar action" (Ayers, 1979, p. 91).

A proprioceptive system that is not sending adequate input to the nervous system can be part of the reason for the "fight or flight" reaction often seen in children with ASD, causing them to be in a hyper-alert state that makes it difficult to feel safe in their bodies (King, 2002b). In order for any kind of learning to take place, the child must be able to notice and feel his body. If the child is anxious about what is happening around her because she does not feel safe in her own body, it is difficult to attend to information – whether new or old (King, 2002b). Table 1.3 list common results of difficulties with the proprioceptive system.

Table 1.3 Challenges Related to the Proprioceptive System	
• Difficulty processing information through proprioceptive system	1. Child does not feel safe in his own body 2. Poor awareness of what his body is doing 3. Contributes to problems with motor planning 4. "Fight or flight" response may become activated

 The Vestibular System

The vestibular system enables us to maintain muscle tone, coordinate both sides of the body, hold our head upright against gravity, coordinate head, eye and body movements, and maintain balance. This system receives information from the inner ear about equilibrium, gravity, movement, and changes of position in space. It is closely related to the auditory system, which has sensory receptors in the inner ear (King, 2002c).

Many children with ASD have difficulty processing information from the vestibular system and may be either over-reactive or under-reactive to vestibular input (Hoekman, 2005). The child who is over-reactive may experience motion sickness in a car or on a swing and may try to avoid excessive movement. In contrast, a child who is under-reactive to vestibular input may be constantly moving, spinning, or flapping. Such a child can have poor balance and frequently bump into things or people. Both of these conditions cause problems with interactions with others as well as joint attention to an activity or event; that is, demonstrating a shared attention to an object or event with another.

Many therapists have observed increased speech production following vestibular stimulation because of the close relationship between the auditory and the vestibular systems (Ayers, 1979; Yack et al., 2002). For this reason, stimulating the vestibular system can be a good strategy when wanting to promote sound production in a child. Equipment that may be used to stimulate the vestibular system includes a swing, rocking chair, Sit N Spin™, or hammock. Table 1.4 shows challenges related to the vestibular system and common results.

Table 1.4 Challenges Related to the Vestibular System	
• Disorders processing information with the vestibular system	1. Disorganization 2. Low muscle tone 3. Difficulty processing auditory input
• Over-sensitivity in the vestibular receptors	1. Motion sickness/nausea from movement 2. Avoidance of excessive movement 3. Poor balance 4. Fear of movement
• Under-sensitivity in the vestibular receptors	1. Constant movement or spinning 2. Poor balance 3. Hyperactivity and distractibility 4. Tendency to bump into people or objects, standing too close to others

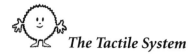 *The Tactile System*

The tactile or touch system refers to the receptors in the skin that send stimulation to the central nervous system. Stimulation from these receptors registers light touch, pressure touch, as well as heat, cold, and pain (King, 2002a). The tactile system is the first sensory system to develop and is needed for development and survival (Yack et al., 2002).

Children with ASD often exhibit excessive sensitivity to touch (Field, 2001). This is the most common symptom of an immature tactile system, and is referred to as tactile hypersensitivity. Examples include the infant or child crying when being picked up and avoidance of shampooing, washing, hair brushing, and tooth brushing. Feeding and speech problems can also result from sensitivity in and around the mouth, as will be explored in more depth later on.

Due to excessive sensitivity to touch, the child is constantly on the alert, making it difficult for him to attend to input coming from the environment through any of the other sensory systems. That is, the child has difficulty paying attention to anything else until he knows what is touching or might touch him (Hoekman, 2005). This leads to tactile *defensiveness*, which causes the child to react negatively or emotionally to another's touch (Ayers, 1979). The child might cry, rub the area touched, or strike out aggressively. Sustained firm pressure and even touch that is maintained for a short time period can help to reduce hyper-reaction or over-reaction to touch.

Children can also be under-reactive to touch, referred to as *tactile hyposensitivity*, which causes an intense need to touch everything or a lack of desire to touch anything that is not familiar (Hoekman, 2005). They may need intense input in order to register the touch. These children don't get information about where they are being touched, which inhibits body awareness and interferes with motor planning. Hyposensitivity to touch can also impede oral movements during eating and speech production (Yack et al., 2002).

In addition, over the course of the day, the tactile system may change due to varying sensory experiences. For example, light touch, such as the wind blowing on the child's face, can be too much tactile input to process on one day but not on another. This is due to the amount of sensory information that the child has had to process prior to the wind touching his face. It is important to understand this when interacting with a child who has become overstimulated for what seems to be unknown reasons. Table 1.5 illustrates reactions to challenges related to the tactile system.

Table 1.5 Challenges Related to the Tactile System	
• Disorders processing information through the tactile system	1. Might react defensively to touch from others 2. Motor planning problems
• Hypersensitive to touch	1. Overly sensitive to touch 2. Avoids having teeth brushed, hair washed/brushed, and face washed 3. Feeding problems, including sensitivities to food textures and temperatures 4. Poor use of lips and tongue 5. On alert, making it difficult to attend in the classroom
• Hyposensitive to touch	1. Seeks excessive amounts of touch stimulation 2. Over-stuffs mouth; messy eater 3. Unaware of build-up of saliva in the mouth, causing drooling 4. Poor use of lips and tongue

Muscle Tone

The neurological system determines our level of muscle tone. Sound muscle tone enables us to keep our bodies in position and gives us the ability to move. Muscle tone is the dynamic state of the body musculature in preparation for movement. It reflects the reactions of the central nervous system to sensory input. It is a state of readiness, which is the result of a normal cycle of sensory-motor-sensory impulses. For example, if you try to straighten someone's arm, the muscles will quickly contract in response, but then relax after the stimulus has ended (Gagnon, 2003).

Muscle tone provides a normal physical structure with its various degrees of stability and mobility. This enables a child to sit in a chair while listening to instruction without fear of falling over or out of the chair. The child can reach for anything easily on a table or on the floor and sit back upright again. The child is stable, which enables him to easily move against gravity.

What happens if we don't have adequate muscle tone?

High muscle tone. A child with high tone, or hypertonia, overreacts to the stimuli that the person with normal tone handles smoothly. The muscle will react at a faster rate and will recover at a slower rate, which creates a lack of readiness for dynamic movement. Children with high muscle tone are often described as stiff or spastic in their movements (Gagnon, 2003). They have difficulty sitting upright in a chair without special adaptations such as a strap across the lap. It might also be difficult for them to hold their head up against gravity or reach for something without falling over.

This is where compensations can begin to occur. For example, the child might hold her head back on her shoulders, causing the muscles at the back of the head to become even more restricted in order to hold the head up against gravity. Further, the rigidity of the muscles makes it difficult for the child's body to be stable, which interferes with the ability to move.

Table 1.6 Hypertonia	
• High muscle tone/hypertonia	1. The muscles react at a faster rate and recover at a slower rate 2. Stiff or spastic movements 3. Difficulty sitting upright in a chair without special adaptations 4. Compensatory movement patterns such as holding head back on shoulders to keep it up against gravity

Low muscle tone. In children with low muscle tone, or hypotonia, on the other hand, the muscles are slow to initiate a contraction and do not fully contract. Often these children also have difficulty maintaining the contraction for as long as someone with normal muscle tone. Low muscle tone causes muscles to be floppy (Gagnon, 2003). Children with hypotonia may also have difficulty sitting upright in a chair. You might observe the child laying her head and body on the table because it is difficult to hold them upright against gravity. The child might even prefer to lie on the floor and resist sitting in a chair during classroom instruction.

Table 1.7 Hypotonia	
• Low muscle tone/hypotonia	1. The muscles are slow to initiate a contraction and do not fully contract 2. Floppy movements 3. Needs a chair with supports 4. May prefer to lie on the floor rather than sit

Further, children with low muscle tone may have difficulty initiating movement at a normal rate and maintain movement. They may be slow to respond to sensory input, have difficulty maintaining a response, and may need physical support from their environment. Support from the environment could be a chair with arm supports and at a height where the feet can be firmly planted on the floor. With this the children can be in a stable position, sitting upright with their body in the middle and in a position to produce the best movements that are possible for them. Our bodies move best when there is stability, with the body centered and balanced at midline.

Dysarthria

Dysarthria is a term used to describe poor control of the speech musculature due to muscle weakness, an inability to use force when moving the muscles, slowness to respond, or incoordination. This can vary in severity from mild to severe. This weakness is due to damage to the central nervous system, the peripheral nervous system, or both (Beckman, 1995a). Dysarthria can cause problems with the control needed to develop oral-motor skills, feeding skills, and speech production. It causes weak, imprecise, and arhythmical movements (Rehabilitation Institute of Chicago, 2002). This can interfere with the child's ability to produce vowel sounds during cooing, consonant-vowel combinations during babbling, complex sound combinations during jargoning, a stage in development where there are a variety of sounds sequenced with inflection, as well as the production of single words, phrases, and conversational speech. The child's speech production can also be imprecise, slow, and weak, causing it to sound slurred.

Further, dysarthria can affect the ability to maintain breath support, vocal quality, and prosody (Rehabilitation Institute of Chicago, 2002). Prosody is the combination of intonation, stress patterns, loudness variations, pausing, and rhythm that is expressed by varying pitch, loudness, and duration. A child with dysarthria can have a rate of speech that is too fast or too slow, a breathy, harsh or hoarse vocal quality, or an excessively loud or soft volume level all due to poor control.

Dysarthria may be manifested in different ways in individual children. For example, the child might have difficulty initiating oral movements for eating or speech production or coordinating the oral movement with the initiation of voice. The dysarthria may cause a vocal pattern that sounds "robotic" or lacking intonation, a term that is sometimes used to describe the speech pattern of some children with ASD (Rapin, 1997). Dysarthria affects many or all of the basic aspects of eating and speech production (Beckman, 1995a).

Table 1.8 Dysarthria	
• Dysarthria	1. Poor control of the speech musculature 2. Weak, imprecise, and arhythmical movements 3. Slurred speech production 4. Difficulty controlling rate, loudness levels, and vocal pitch and quality 5. Difficulty with initiation of voice 6. Difficulty swallowing, sucking, and chewing

Apraxia

Apraxia is a disorder of motor-speech programming (Murdoch, Ozanne, & Cross, 1990). Apraxia of speech, or verbal apraxia, refers to the inability to voluntarily combine, organize, and sequence movements necessary to produce clear and precise speech. It is a sensory-motor disorder that can cause difficulty programming and planning speech movements (Kumin, 2002).

In typical development, the child listens to speech sounds in the environment and then practices the sounds during cooing, babbling, and jargoning. The child develops a feedback system for producing the sounds quickly, and the production of these sound sequences becomes automatic through experience and practice (Kumin, 2002).

Verbal apraxia. The child with verbal apraxia, by contrast, cannot integrate all the incoming sensory-motor information, making it difficult to develop a feedback system for producing sounds quickly. He may have been a quiet baby who did not frequently coo or babble. According to Ayers (1979), it is difficult to develop complex movement patterns, such as connected speech, when you cannot organize and plan simple movements due to a poor sense of your body. As we have seen earlier, this can occur due to poor registering of sensory information, difficulty modulating sensory input, and an inability and lack of motivation to initiate movements, all of which have found to be characteristics of children with autism (Yack et al., 2002). Many children with a diagnosis of ASD exhibit verbal apraxia.

Some characteristics of verbal apraxia include inconsistent errors of speech, a limited repertoire of speech sounds due to multiple articulation errors, an uneven rhythm of speech production, and difficulty combining and sequencing speech sounds, especially as the words become longer and more complex (Lucker-Lazerson, 2003).

Table 1.9 Verbal Apraxia	
• Verbal apraxia	1. An inability to combine, organize, and sequence movements needed for speech production, especially as words become complex 2. A "quiet baby" who did not play with sounds 3. Inconsistent speech errors 4. An uneven speech rhythm 5. A limited quantity of speech sounds 6. Multiple articulation errors

Oral apraxia. Different from verbal apraxia, oral apraxia involves difficulty with the production of volitional oral movements such as sticking out the tongue or licking one's lips even when otherwise capable of producing these movements (Apraxia-Kids, 2005). For example, a child with oral apraxia may be observed licking his lips while eating but be unable to do this movement when asked to "lick your lips" or "do this."

Table 1.10 Oral Apraxia	
• Oral apraxia	1. Difficulty with producing oral movements when asked 2. Can produce oral movements spontaneously while eating or playing

Dysarthria vs. Apraxia

The same child can exhibit oral apraxia, verbal apraxia, and dysarthria to varying degrees. In fact, it is more common for these disorders to occur together than in isolation. For example, a child whose primary disability is verbal apraxia can exhibit oral apraxia and a mild level of dysarthria. Children with severe dysarthria can also have verbal apraxia.

The apraxia might not be observed until after the child is able to produce speech sounds. Prior to that, the muscle weakness and incoordination might have been the primary disability. The dysarthria can also make it difficult to produce volitional oral movements, which would hinder a diagnosis of oral apraxia. For example, due to muscle weakness and incoordination, the child cannot elevate all the muscles of the tongue together for a tongue click. It is difficult to observe the child's ability to motor plan this movement until he can produce it on an automatic level as should be the case in apraxia (Murdoch et al., 1990).

The oral-motor program presented in Chapter 3 will assist in developing oral awareness and a feedback system for producing oral movements. "One may postulate that if feedback is enhanced, subsequent movements may be improved" (Redstone, 2007, p. 121). It will enhance the child's ability to integrate and respond to tactile input around and inside of the mouth. This, in turn, will enable the child to better imitate, produce, and sequence oral movements for eating and speech production.

Delayed vs. Disordered Development

Children with ASD often exhibit both delayed and disordered development. The term *delayed development* indicates that the child is developing the same skills as her typical peers but at a slower rate. An example would be the child who continues to primarily explore objects by mouthing past 15 months of age. This child would be delayed in the ability to interact/explore objects, which affects her ability to see the differences between objects. Children with ASD may continue to mouth longer than is typical because of an immature tactile system, causing them to crave more tactile input (Yack et al., 2002). Further, primitive patterns can also be observed with children with ASD. These are patterns seen during the first four months of development, such as the oral reflexes (Bobath & Bobath, 1975; Evans-Morris & Dunn-Klein, 1987).

Disordered development* or *abnormal development, on the other hand, refers to skills or behaviors that would not be seen in the child's typical peers (Bobath & Bobath, 1975). They may be compensations for the child's sensory-motor disorder. For example, some children with ASD are not able to look at the person they are interacting with at a particular moment. They may not be able to listen and look at the same time because their system is on sensory overload. Their way to compensate for this would be to look away while they are attempting to listen or talk.

An example of an abnormal movement is a tongue thrust. The tongue has a thick or bunched appearance and moves forcefully over the lower lip. This could occur while drinking from a cup where the tongue is thrust into or underneath the cup (Beckman, 1995b).

Summary

The information in this chapter is necessary to understand the reasons behind the development of the treatment environment, the prescribed usage of language, and the oral-motor treatment program presented in Chapter 3. Also, the terms common to this diagnosis are frequently heard during the evaluation process and need to be understood by both parents and teachers. Parents and teachers need to understand why the child is behaving in a certain manner. The behaviors associated with processing disorders in the different sensory systems were described to assist with this. ■

X

CHAPTER 2

Evaluation of Oral-Motor Development

This chapter presents an overview of typical child development and the process of evaluating oral-motor development. It is essential to know typical development to be able to identify when someone is exhibiting delayed, primitive, abnormal, or disordered development. For that reason, the speech-language pathologist evaluating a child must have extensive knowledge of typical development. Parents and teachers also should be knowledgeable about this area so that they will know when it is appropriate to refer a child for an evaluation or at least make inquiries.

Included in this chapter are descriptions of normal and abnormal oral development. Most important, is a description of what the evaluator should be observing and what some of these observations might indicate for a given child.

Typical Development

Many children with autism spectrum disorders (ASD) demonstrate delayed, primitive, and/or abnormal oral-motor development, which impacts their speech and expressive language development as well as their eating development. Some behaviors that suggest the need for an evaluation of the child's oral-motor skills by a licensed speech-language pathologist with knowledge about normal and abnormal oral-motor development include:

- Excessive food loss/messiness while eating

- Mouthing inedible objects after age 2

- Presence of oral reflexes after 8 months of age

- Excessive drooling

- Unintelligible speech production after age 3

Note. The book *Pre-Feeding Skills* by Suzanne Evans-Morris, Ph.D., C.C.C., and Marsha Dunn-Klein, M.Ed., O.T.R. (1987) is a good reference for this kind of information.

Table 2.1 shows a brief overview of normal oral-motor, feeding, and speech/language development, including how the child's oral-motor skills, feeding skills, and speech skills develop together. Normal development begins at birth and occurs from head to toe. The oral muscles are some of the first muscles that the child is able to use. This is seen in Table 2.1 under 0 to 3 months, where the child has function with the oral structures through the oral reflexes. For example, the head and tongue move reflexively in the newborn during the rooting reflex in an attempt to find the mother's nipple for nourishment.

By reviewing Table 2.1, teachers and parents can get a general idea of whether the skills exhibited by the child are within normal limits or are delayed.

Table 2.1
Typical Oral-Motor/Feeding/Speech/Language Development

0 to 3 months:
- The child uses reflexive/stereotypic movements that are the foundation for later movements. These include the rooting reflex, phasic bite reflex, gag reflex, and suckle-swallow reflex.
- There are forward/backward tongue movements with a flat, cupped tongue configuration to allow for movement of the liquid to the back of the mouth.
- Movements are smooth, easily initiated, and rhythmical. The jaw, lips, and tongue move together as one unit.
- The child produces primarily nasal vowel sounds as air is directed through the nose.
- Head control and midline orientation begin to develop.

4 to 6 months:
- The oral reflexes become integrated.
- A suckling pattern (forward/backward movement) predominates, but there is a beginning of the sucking pattern (up/down movement).
- The center portion of the lips becomes active on nipple.
- The suck/swallow is poorly coordinated with breathing.
- Mouth movements increase due to stability at base of tongue and increased space within the mouth. The tongue no longer fills the mouth.
- The child begins to produce an increase in the variety and amount of sounds, especially with increased movement of the tongue and play with hands to mouth. Sound production is influenced by body position and movements. The child produces back, throaty sounds when lying on her back, lip sounds (m and b) when lying on her stomach, and tongue sounds (d and n) when sitting.

7 to 9 months:
- The rooting reflex has become integrated but may still be seen in breast-fed babies or when the child is fatigued.
- The gag reflex has diminished and become more adult like.
- There is active separate lip movement while cleaning the spoon, on the nipple, and drawing inward of the lower lip with spoon removal.
- The child begins to produce a tongue lag during swallow. This gives the first sensation of the tongue moving separately from the jaw.
- There is no liquid loss with the bottle/breast but still may be seen with a cup due to up/down jaw movement while cup drinking. The child may bite on the cup to stabilize the jaw.
- Jaw stability with solids is beginning as seen through the use of a bite/hold on solid food.
- The child is able to move food from the center of the tongue to the side gums due to the development of independent tongue movements and trunk rotation in sitting.
- The child develops trunk control and sitting balance, which enables him to produce speech sounds separate from movements of the body. However, there continues to be sound production while the child is moving. There is an increase in long strings of repetitive sound production. The child may produce his first word at 9 months.

Table 2.1 (continued)

10 to 12 months:
- The primary movement while eating and drinking is sucking (up/down movement of the tongue).
- There are long sequences of drinking with the bottle/breast.
- The child is able to swallow semi-solids with lip closure and no food loss.
- There is now a controlled sustained bite through a soft cookie, indicating continued increase in jaw stability.
- The child plays with producing different sounds, pitches, and intonations.
- The child is able to produce long strings of a variety of speech sounds and word approximations and gains continued stability and mobility with the gradual increase of postural control against gravity.

13 to 15 months:
- The child continues to stabilize the cup by biting on the edge but is able to move the upper lip downward onto the cup while drinking.
- There is no coughing with drinking from a cup, but the child may produce liquid loss with removal of the cup.
- The lower jaw does not move while the tongue moves to the side teeth.
- The child's body is more stable, which can be seen in ability to walk. At this same time of overall increased stability, the child has developed separate tongue and lip movements from lower jaw movements.
- The child continues to produce long sequences of a variety of sounds with varying intonation patterns. Some describe this as expressive jabbering. There continues to be an increase in single-word production.

16 to 18 months:
- The child uses up/down tongue movement with minimal forward/backward tongue movement for the swallow.
- The child is able to produce a controlled, sustained bite through a hard cookie and is able to chew with lips closed. Some food or saliva loss may occur while chewing.
- The child begins to use the end of the tongue while moving the food to the side teeth, indicating the first separation of one part of the tongue from the other. The use of the end of the tongue is important for speech production.
- The child imitates new sound patterns and single words. The child may have a vocabulary of 5 to 10 words.

19 to 24 months:
- The child no longer needs to bite on the cup and is able to hold the cup edge out on the lower lip while drinking. The child also begins to drink from a straw.
- The child freely moves the tongue in and out while cleaning the lips with skillful movement of the tongue tip independently of jaw movement.
- A forward/backward movement of the tongue may still be seen while swallowing liquids but not with solids or semi-solids.
- The child produces the entire range of vowels and consonants during sound play.
- The child's vocabulary is greatly increased, with a greater variety of word types and meanings. By 24 months, the child typically begins to combine two words.

Table 2.1 (continued)

25 to 36 months:
- The child's oral-pharyngeal anatomy becomes more adult-like.
- The child is able to swallow one portion of solid food while maintaining other solid food in the mouth for further chewing.
- The child can bite through most foods with graded jaw movements and the appropriate amount of mouth opening.
- There is circular, rotary jaw movement while the food is moved side to side in the mouth. The child is also able to move food to either side when requested to do so. When necessary, the child uses lip closure while chewing. A forward tongue movement is no longer seen during the swallow.
- There is no drooling during fine-motor tasks or speech production.
- There is consistency in the production of speech sounds and an increase in the speed of speech production, showing more precise control. By 36 months, the child should be understood by most people even when the topic of conversation is not known.

Note. This overview of typical development is based on information from numerous sources, including Alexander, Boehme, and Cupps (1982) and Evans-Morris and Dunn-Klein (1987).

What to Look For

Initially, during the evaluation, the therapist asks for significant medical or developmental history about the child. This includes prenatal/birth history, feeding or eating history, the child's general health history and development, school history, as well as the results of any testing information and/or reports from prior therapies. The parents are also interviewed during this process because they know their child best (Evans-Morris & Dunn-Klein, 1987). Further, a sensory history and profile will help to identify target behaviors and the situations in which they occur. Parents are often provided with a checklist to fill out prior to the evaluation (Yack et al., 2002).

As part of the evaluation, the child's oral structures are observed at rest, while eating, and during the production of speech. The oral structures observed include the lips, the gums, the jaw, the tongue, the cheeks, the teeth, and the hard and soft palate. While eating, the child is, at a minimum, asked to drink a liquid, eat a semi-solid from a spoon, and chew a solid. Speech production can be observed during formal testing and during conversational speech production.

The oral musculature used by the child for feeding is also used for speech production. Even though the oral movements needed for eating are more basic and automatic than the more complex movement patterns needed for speech production, it is important to observe how the musculature is performing while the child is eating to make sure the components of movement necessary for speech production are also being produced. In other words, the child is producing sensory-motor patterns while eating that are similar to the sensory-motor patterns needed for speech production.

Table 2.2 **Oral Structures**
1. Lips
2. Gums
3. Tongue
4. Cheeks
5. Jaw
6. Palate (hard and soft)
7. Teeth

The child's movements of the oral structures at rest, while eating, and during speech production are described as (a) within normal limits, (b) delayed or primitive, or (c) not developing typically. Also noted at this time are overall muscle tone, body symmetry, body stability and mobility, and coordination of the child's movements through space (see Chapter 1).

The Oral-Motor/Eating/Speech Checklist in Table 2.3 (a blank copy may be found in the Appendix) is an example of a checklist that can be used by the speech-language pathologist to establish a baseline of skills prior to beginning the oral-motor program. This can then be completed again after a period of time to chart the progress made by the child from using the oral-motor program.

Table 2.3
Sample Oral-Motor/Eating/Speech Checklist

Name: _____

Birthdate: _____

Age: _____

Date: _____

I. **Oral Structures/Musculature During Movement**
    I: (imitation)   S: (spontaneous)
    (*Note: asymmetries, movement patterns, and ability to produce separate movements*)

    1. Open mouth: _S_____
    2. Close mouth: S_____
    3. Smile: S greater movement on the right side _____
    4. Pucker: I_____
    5. Blow: I_____
    6. Hum: I, poor lip contact_____
    7. Oo-ee: I, less retraction on the left_____
    8. Lip smack: S_____
    9. Puff out cheeks: unable to do_____
    10. Tongue out (with mouth open): S, tongue pulls to right, wide mouth opening
    11. Tongue out/in (with mouth open): I, tongue pulls to the right, wide mouth opening
    12. Tongue tip up inside of mouth: unable to do_____
    13. Tongue tip to upper lip: unable to do_____
    14. Tongue tip down inside of mouth: unable to do_____
    15. Tongue tip to lower lip: I_____
    16. Tongue side to side to mouth corners: I, to the right side but not to the left side, jaw follows
    17. Tongue side to side to lower teeth: I, to the right side but not to the left side, jaw follows
    18. Tongue side to side to cheeks: I, to the right side but not to the left side, jaw follows
    19. Tongue side to side to upper teeth: unable to do____
    20. Tongue click: I, jaw and tongue move together_____
    21. Click teeth: I_____

II. **Oral and Postural Muscle Tone**
    1. Facial tone: low muscle tone_____
    2. Lingual tone: low muscle tone_____
    3. Body tone: low muscle tone_____

Table 2.3 (continued)

III. Respiration

1. Oral breather: _maintains open mouth_
2. Nasal breather: _____

IV. Movements While Eating

1. Food texture prefer: _crunchy solids_
2. Food texture avoid: _slimy texture_
3. Description of movements with:

   A. liquid: _liquid loss_

       a. cup: _forward/backward tongue movement, bites on cup edge_

       b. straw: _drinks out of right side of mouth_

   B. semi-solid from a spoon: _poor lip closure on the spoon,_
   forward/backward tongue movement during the swallow

   C. soft solid: _chews with wide vertical movements_

   D. hard solid: _refuses_

V. Vocal Quality

1. Normal: _+_
2. Breathy: _____
3. Harsh: _____
4. Hoarse: _____
5. Nasal: _____
6. De-nasal: _____
7. High pitch: _____
8. Low or high volume level: _____

VI. Speech-Language Production

1. Sound play: _____
2. Gestures/sign language: _____
3. Sound imitation: _____
4. Word imitation: _I, single words, tongue, lips, and jaw move together_
5. Word production: _S, single words, tongue, lips, and jaw move together_
6. Production of phrases: _unable to do_
7. Sentence length/complexity: _unable to do_
8. Low or high volume level: _poor volume control, either very quiet or very loud_

Due to his/her extensive knowledge of normal development, the speech-language pathologist will be able to diagnose the child's movement patterns and explain these as normal, delayed, primitive, or abnormal/disordered (Beckman, 1995b; Bobath & Bobath 1975). The information given here is meant to enable parents and teachers to have a brief overview of the evaluation process so they know what to expect from the professionals working with their child.

Results of Evaluation

Delayed Development

As mentioned in Chapter 1, the child's movements are delayed if he produces movements that are typically seen in normal development but at a younger age. An example of a child with a delayed oral-motor skill would be the child who is 3 years of age or older and who continues to bite on the cup edge while drinking, a behavior that is seen in normal development but at a younger age. Typically, the child aged 24 months (see Table 2.1) no longer needs to bite on the cup while drinking because he has developed internal jaw stability (Evans-Morris & Dunn Klein, 1987). A child who continues to bite on the cup past 24 months, therefore, would have delayed oral-motor/eating skills due to a lack of internal jaw control.

The lack of internal jaw control also affects the production of speech and other oral movements. For example, this child would typically move his tongue and jaw together while moving food from side to side rather than moving the tongue separately from the jaw. He might also be difficult to understand when the topic of conversation is not known, due to a lack of independent tongue and lip movement from jaw movement because of a lack of internal jaw control.

The continued presence of the oral reflexes such as the rooting reflex, a food-seeking reflex, or the phasic bite reflex, a rhythmical, food-pumping reflex, after an age when they should be integrated into the child's nervous system (usually between 4 and 6 months of age) would be considered primitive movements. As mentioned in Chapter 1, the term *primitive* is used to refer to movements that are typically only seen in an infant (Bobath &

Bobath, 1975). Primitive movement patterns are listed in Table 2.1 in the birth to 3 months section and the 4 to 6 month section.

Abnormal Development

The child might also produce movements not seen in normal development. These are referred to as abnormal or disordered oral movements. Abnormal or disordered patterns of movement would be present during all oral movements such as eating, purposeful oral movement, and speech production. They may be due to hyper- or hypo-muscle tone, causing the child to compensate to be able to produce purposeful movement (Bobath & Bobath, 1975).

An example would be a tongue thrust where the tongue moves forward out of the mouth. This movement pattern could be the result of abnormal muscle tone causing the muscles of the base of the tongue to become restricted or fixed. The forward tongue movement occurs as the child attempts to move the tongue against this restriction (Beckman, 1995b).

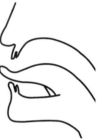

Tongue Thrust

As pointed out in Chapter 1, children with ASD often exhibit low or hypo-muscle tone, which provides a poor base of support for the development of movement. The child must work harder in order to use muscles with low muscle tone (Gagnon, 2003). As the child begins to move against gravity, she begins to fix, or hold abnormally, certain parts of her body to gain stability so movement can occur. As more fixing occurs, normal components of movement are unable to develop. Fixing in one area will result in compensatory movement patterns in other areas, causing abnormal sensory-motor feedback and abnormal responses of the central nervous system.

Another example of an abnormal movement pattern would be tongue retraction, where the tongue is drawn upward and backward in the mouth.

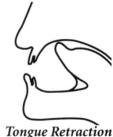

Tongue Retraction

This inhibits the child's ability to actively move the tongue (Beckman, 1995b). The tongue retraction might have developed as the child attempted to hold her head up or open her mouth as a newborn.

Other examples of abnormal movement patterns include jaw retraction and retraction of the cheeks and lips (Beckman, 1995b). With cheek/lip retraction, the cheeks and lips are pulled backward, making it difficult to produce lip closure while eating, during oral movements, and speech production.

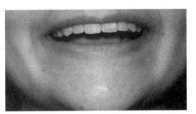

Cheek/Lip Retraction

Asymmetrical movement patterns can also result from fixing in one part of the body. For example, the child's tongue may pull to one side when she is asked, "stick out your tongue," or she may only be able to move food to one side of the mouth.

These atypical movement patterns cause abnormal sensory-motor feedback and abnormal responses of the central nervous system. This in turn interferes with the child's ability to produce adaptive responses and can cause him to over- or an under-react to sensory information. An example would be a hyper-active or hypo-active gag reflex, which could cause the child to become defensive when approached by someone attempting to provide oral input (Watson, 2001). This might be observed during a parent's attempt to brush the child's teeth. Indeed, many parents report tooth brushing is difficult with children with ASD.

Developing a Treatment Plan

Following the oral-motor evaluation, the speech-language pathologist is able to provide families and educators with a description of the child's oral-motor skills and how they are impacting eating and speech/language development. A comprehensive treatment plan can then be developed for the child to facilitate her ability to produce oral movements at her potential, as illustrated in the case of Amy in the following.

Amy, a 4-year-old girl, drank with the cup pushed far back in her mouth, which interfered with her ability to develop jaw control while drinking. She had difficulty moving food side to side in her mouth. Amy often had to rely on head movements to get the food to the side teeth for chewing or just mashed food up against her hard palate prior to swallowing it. Her speech production was hard to understand by most people, sometimes even by her family members.

A treatment plan for Amy must address her oral movements while eating and speaking in order to make changes with all of her skills at an automatic level. Improved head/neck alignment and trunk stability must also be a part of her treatment plan. "Proximal stability can result in better functioning of a distal structure such as the mouth" (Redstone, 2007, p. 124).

The oral-motor program described in Chapter 3 is an essential part of a comprehensive treatment program. It takes into consideration that the child can exhibit delayed, primitive and abnormal movement patterns, hypo-or hyper-muscle tone, verbal apraxia, dysarthria, oral apraxia, and an abnormal sensory-motor feedback system. It presents sensory input in an organized manner so the child can make use of the input and produce more normalized patterns of movement.

Summary

This chapter outlined the role and functions of the speech-language pathologist performing an oral-motor evaluation. In addition, an overview of normal development as it relates to oral-motor, feeding, and speech/language was presented to help parents and teachers gain knowledge about what to expect during the evaluation process. ■

X

CHAPTER 3

Treatment and the Treatment Environment

For children who receive a diagnosis of oral-motor disorder, feeding disorder, motor-speech disorder, or communication disorder following a comprehensive speech/language evaluation, the treatment program presented in this chapter will be beneficial. The program allows the child to make use of the sensory input and produce more normalized patterns of movement. "The goal is to increase the possibility of a more normal motor response through manipulation of the sensory environment" (Alexander, 1987, as cited in Redstone, 2007, p. 125). It can be used at home, in the classroom, or in the therapy room. The treatment environment, oral-motor program, and activities are described in detail here so that parents, teachers, teacher assistants, or other caretakers working with the child can easily carry out the program.

Preparation

Setting up for the Session

Structuring the treatment environment is essential for facilitating a successful session with the child. This chapter gives suggestions on positioning, language usage, and control of background sensory stimulation. Most important, the oral-motor program, a structured, routine series of oral exercises is described in detail so that parents and teachers can easily incorporate it into their daily routines. Also included are lists of materials, activities, and foods that promote mature oral patterns, along with explanations of how and why. Finally, the stages of imitation are defined and described so this essential skill can be enhanced with the child and the communicative partner (Marshalla, 2001).

Seating

Optimally, the child and parent/teacher/therapist are seated facing each other at eye level at a distance of about an arm's length in preparation for the oral-motor exercises. As stated in Chapter 1, children with an autism spectrum disorder (ASD) have difficulty registering tactile input, making it difficult for them to interpret tactile information and causing them to be defensive or on alert (Ayers, 1979). Consequently, it is important to observe the child's reaction and adjust the distance between the two of you if the child becomes defensive while talking about what you are going to be doing together. This may be as simple as just asking, "Can I work with you now?"

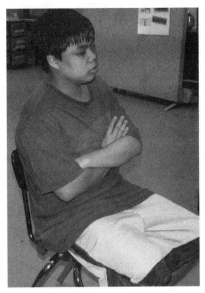

Child sitting at 90-degree angle.

The child should be seated upright in a chair at a 90-degree angle with both feet firmly on the floor (Redstone, 2004). He should not be in a chair where his feet are dangling or his back is slouched against the back of the chair. Since children with ASD often do not get accurate feedback from their proprioceptive system as to where their body is in space (Ayers, 1979), it is important that they are in a stable position so that they can focus on what they are doing rather than on how they are going to stay in the chair. Also, as we have seen in Chapter 2, low muscle tone makes it difficult to maintain postural control because the muscles do not fully contract and remain floppy (Gagnon, 2003). This is another reason to make sure that the child is in a stable position prior to beginning work.

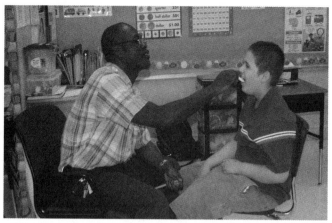

Child and therapist/parent facing each other during oral-motor program.

An alternative to a regular chair is a beanbag chair. This surrounds the child and helps give her feedback as to where her body is in space. This postural control in turn enhances the child's ability to produce active movement. In short, a stable sitting position can improve oral-motor skills.

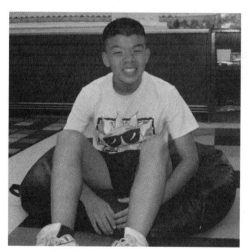

Child sitting in bean bag chair.

General Environment

The environment should be relatively quiet and without a lot of visual stimulation. This helps the child pay attention to you. The child may be unable to filter out background stimuli, making it difficult to attend to the most important information.

On a day where the child has reached the limit for what information or stimulation she can process, she might need to shut out all other sensory information. This can cause an unacceptable response or no response at all. For example, the child might sit or lie down on the floor with her head down and eyes closed, unable to respond to questions or comments from others. These responses can occur without much warning and seem variable or difficult to interpret since we don't always know everything that has occurred to the child over the course of the day. For these reasons, it is important to present sensory information in an organized manner with minimum background stimulation.

Language Use

How language is presented to the child is part of the treatment environment. The adult's language is a component of the sensory information processed by the child. It needs to be presented in an organized and simple fashion so the child can process and use the information without becoming overwhelmed and overstimulated. As mentioned, the child's tolerance can change on a day-to-day basis depending on the amount of information he has been exposed to over the course of the day and what else has been going on around him.

1. **In presenting the oral-motor program to the child, use language consisting of simple sentence structure that is grammatically accurate.** Since children with ASD can become overwhelmed with auditory input (Rapin, 1997), it is important to ensure that information is correct and at a minimum. A slow rate of speech with a pause after each sentence will also help with the child's auditory processing

skills. Observe the child's face and body to make sure that she is attending to what you have said to her. You should be at eye level. If possible, ask the child to repeat the comment or direction back to ensure that he has processed the information.

2. **Start the session with the same phrase each time so the child knows what to expect.** For example, "It is time for oral-motor. Get your oral-motor bag." The language that you use while doing the oral-motor techniques should also stay relatively the same. When the language stays the same, the child can learn the script and use the language to respond, comment, initiate, or request. For example, the person working with the child could say, "It is time for your _____." The child, knowing the routine, would know to respond with "Nuk brush." The Nuk brush could also be held up at this time to give the child an added visual cue to the correct response.

   Also, understanding what usually happens next enables the child to accurately follow directions during the oral-motor time. This helps him to become independent within group time. The child is able to "put away the chew tube and get out the Nuk brush" without assistance from an adult or the visual cue.

3. **Tell the child what is going to happen and what is happening throughout all the exercises and activities.** Children with ASD have difficulty interpreting nonverbal cues and have atypical, defensive tactile systems (Ayers, 1979). If they do not understand what is going to happen or what is happening, the "fight or flight" reflex may be elicited, causing them to withdraw or become aggressive. Specific language, such as, "It is time to touch your face now," may help the child know what to expect. This information can be repeated to assist with auditory processing.

In summary, using specific language will help the child tolerate touch and avoid negative behaviors by helping him to anticipate what will happen next. Since his tactile system makes it difficult to modulate touch from others, this will help to inhibit emotional, over-reactions to touch (Ayers, 1979).

Oral-Motor Box/Bag

The oral-motor bag/box (see Table 3.1) should have the child's name on it and should be kept at school and at home. Plan a regular oral-motor time at school as part of the child's schedule. This may be before lunch or a lesson where the child is expected to produce verbal language.

At home, the oral-motor bag or box may be given to the child when she appears to need oral stimulation such as when she puts inedible objects or fingers in her mouth. It may also be used when there is an overall need for some kind of an activity, such as when the child has become overstimulated and needs to calm down, or at a regularly scheduled time. Many of the materials typically included in an oral-motor bag/box may be bought at a grocery or discount store or ordered from a catalogue specializing in speech and oral-motor materials (see the resource section of the Appendix).

Table 3.1 Typical Contents of Oral-Motor Box/Bag
• A variety of toothbrushes
• Mini massager
• Flavored tongue depressors
• Chew tubes
• Flavored gloves
• Variety of whistles and hum-a-zoos
• Flavor sprays
• Bubbles
• Lollipops
• ChapStick®
• Washcloths
• Lotion
• Powder
• Powder puffs
• Hand mitts
• Oral-motor playing cards

Treatment

The oral-motor program introduced here is based on predictable tactile input presented in a manner that is acceptable to the child. In this way, the child can use the input to develop a sense of self and can grow and develop new skills. It is best if the treatment activities are performed prior to a meal, snack, purposeful movement, or verbal routines since the child's system has then been prepared for better oral function and the development of a more normalized feedback system. That is, the child can now better interpret and monitor her oral tactile information and can receive "feedback" from her tactile system on how she is moving her oral structures. This helps her remember the movement patterns so that she can produce them again at a later time in a similar situation.

Touch is an important way for us to experience the world around us. Touch is the first sensory system to develop, and it is important for survival, learning, self-esteem, growth, and development. Children with ASD are often aversive to touch (Field, 2001), which makes it difficult for them to use this sense to experience their world and develop a sense of themselves. They become on the alert, impeding their ability to process new information for learning and continued development.

Benefits of Organized Touch

A study (Escalona, Field, Singer-Strunch, Cullen, & Hartshorn, 2001) with preschool-aged children who had a diagnosis of autism focused on the benefits of organized touch. The children were given a massage for a 10-day period. After the 10 days, the children's ability to relate to their teachers increased, and their disruptive behaviors in the classroom setting decreased.

In another study (Escalona et al., 2001), parents were taught to massage their children, who had a diagnosis of autism, each night. The researchers found that these children experienced the same benefits as in the first study as well as increased amounts of sleep. The researchers speculated that the children accepted the massage because it was predictable tactile input. Similarly, Ackerman (1991, as cited in Yack et al., 2002) found that premature infants who receive consistent massage are more alert, active, and calm with better orienting responses.

The feet, palms of the hand, fingertips, tongue, lips and face have more touch-sensitive nerve cells than other parts of the body (Field, 2001). Predictable touch stimulation to areas of the body that have increased touch-sensitive nerve cells can cause general relaxation in the body and a more attentive state (Field, 2001). For this reason, these parts of the body are addressed in a structured, predictable manner in the oral-motor program presented here.

The child is encouraged to participate with the tactile activities and exercises but is never forced to do so. Forcing would increase the "fight or flight" response and interfere with the purpose of using tactile input to facilitate automatic movement patterns and sensory responses.

1. **Have the child apply lotion.** The children are encouraged to rub the lotion first by themselves with firm touch. Since children with ASD often have tactile defensiveness, they are better able to accept this tactile input when provided by themselves (Ayers, 1979). They begin with one leg and foot before moving to the other leg and foot. They then rub the lotion on one arm and one hand and then the other arm and hand. Finally, they rub the lotion on their face. The child's body is being prepared to accept tactile stimulation inside the mouth and to be in a more relaxed, alert state.

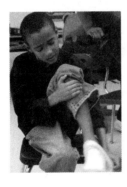 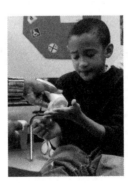 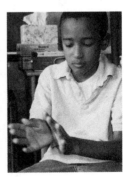

Getting ready for group. *Putting on the lotion.* *Rubbing lotion on hands.*

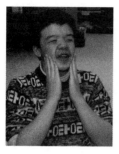 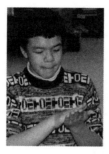 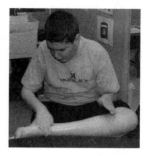

Rubbing lotion on face.   *Rubbing lotion on hands.*   *Rubbing lotion on legs.*

While they are rubbing lotion on the face, encourage the children to rub in the direction of the mouth and down along the side of the lower jaw line. It is important to watch the size of the mouth opening while the child is rubbing lotion on his face. This is a good time to encourage the child to *grade the size* of his mouth—control the size of the mouth opening. For example, say "make your mouth small," "make your lips touch," or "close your mouth."

Sometimes children need assistance with rubbing lotion on their face and body or with grading the size of their mouth. Ask for permission, prior to assisting with rubbing in the lotion. For example, "Can I help you rub the lotion?" or "Can I touch your face?" Carefully watch the child's reaction to make sure your touch is acceptable. Help rub the lotion or support the jaw by placing a hand or finger under the child's chin and your index finger under the lower lip. It is important to use firm touch since this is easier to tolerate than light touch (Genna, 2001).

While rubbing each part of the body with lotion, you can help the child verbally describe what he is doing. For example, "I am rubbing my leg." This may also be sung. The song "This is the way I rub my _____" works well while the children are rubbing lotion on themselves. When the same words and the same order of words are used each time, the child is more likely to actively participate in the activity because he is able to predict what to do and say next.

This predictable order also assists with teaching the names of the body parts. Due to difficulty registering, modulating, and interpreting tactile and auditory information, children might not be able to identify and name their body parts. In this way children are learning the names of the body parts while improving tactile discrimination and developing a feedback system. It also prepares them to tolerate input on the lips and inside of the mouth. Finally, the predictable tactile input given to the body and face can cause a generalized state of relaxation throughout the body and reduce tactile defensiveness (Genna, 2001).

2. **Have the child provide tactile stimulation to her lips.** It is important to focus on the lips because of the large number of touch-sensitive nerve cells in that area. Children can use a flavored ChapStick®, rub their lips with a soft cloth, or touch their lips with firm pressure. It is important to help them describe what they are doing. For example, "I am touching my lips" or "I am rubbing ChapStick on my lips."

3. **Ask the child, "get your chew tube."** Consistent use of the chew tube will assist with developing jaw stability, which is needed for the progression of separate tongue and lip movement to occur.

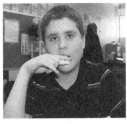
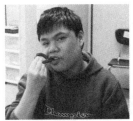
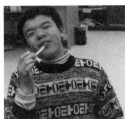

Using T-shaped chew tube. *Using P-shaped chew tube.* *Using T-shaped chew tube.*

Encourage the child to chew in a continuous, rhythmical manner for 10 to 30 times on each side of the mouth. Count out loud, sometimes with clapping, to assist with developing a rhythm. Count the same number each time so the child knows what to expect. The child can then verbally or nonverbally participate in counting the chews on each side.

This is another time when the child can be encouraged to grade the size of the mouth opening. The child's mouth should not be fully extended while chewing. Assist by placing a hand or finger under the child's chin with thumb under the lower lip to facilitate a smaller mouth opening (Redstone, 2004).

You may also ask the child to "make his mouth smaller" while chewing. Make sure that the child's jaw is moving up and down, and not to either side or forward. Again, by placing a hand under the child's chin, you will give the lower jaw support and help it to stay in midline. If this does not help to keep the child's jaw in the middle, finish with the chew tube for that session. It does not help the child to practice chewing with the jaw moving side to side or forward. Try the chew tube again the next time.

4. **Instruct the child to "put away your chew tube and get your Nuk brush."** The Nuk brush is a massage brush originally designed for infants, but frequently used by therapists to increase oral awareness and improve oral sensitivity. "Put away your chew tube and get your Nuk brush" is a two-step direction that the child is likely to follow because she is familiar with the routine. It is important to emphasize that the Nuk brush is not meant to be chewed.

The child pushes down on her tongue with the Nuk brush while the tongue is inside of the mouth. This will help facilitate the development of tongue movement separate from jaw movement and increase awareness. If there is no separation of tongue movement from jaw movement, the child will have trouble keeping her tongue in her mouth with the mouth open. Support at the lower jaw will help keep the mouth open. The child is encouraged to push down on the front half of the tongue for 10 to 30 times with the adult counting out loud while the tongue is inside of the mouth. This is to increase awareness of the body of the tongue while inside of the mouth and to assist in developing normal oral sensitivity (Clark, 2006; Lazarus, 2006; Sheppard, 2006). Continue to

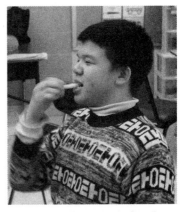

Using a Nuk massage brush on the tongue.

encourage the child to "keep a small mouth" while pushing down on her tongue with the Nuk brush.

The child next brushes both sides of the tongue. This encourages tongue movement separate from the lower jaw to the side teeth. The child also brushes the front third of the top of the mouth. Remind him to move the tongue up to the top of the mouth by first touching the front of the tongue and then the top of the mouth. Also do this with the end or tip of the tongue. Encourage the child to push down on the end of the tongue and then touch the top of the mouth behind the upper teeth. Typically, the tongue will

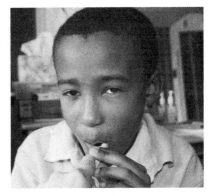

Using a Nuk massage brush on the side of the tongue.

follow the tactile stimulation and move to the top of the mouth. All these activities with the Nuk brush are meant to encourage tongue movement independent of jaw movement and to assist in normalizing oral sensitivity (Clark, 2006; Lazarus, 2006; Sheppard, 2006).

Tongue strengthening exercises that encourage movement against resistance may also be used at this time (Logemann, 2006). Case studies (Clark, 2006; Lazarus, 2006; Sheppard, 2006) have examined the effect of isometric exercises (strength training exercises) (Anderson, 2001) and found them to be effective in improving tongue strength, muscle tone, and swallow function.

The parent, teacher, or therapist pushes down on the front of the child's tongue while the tongue is inside the mouth. The child is encouraged to push up against this resistance to the top of the mouth. This can be done 5 to 10 times. This same exercise may also be done with the end or tip of the tongue.

The oral-program data sheet (see Table 3.2) can be used to keep track of the child's responses to the use of lotion, ChapStick, chew tube, and Nuk brush on a daily basis. Following is an example of an oral-motor program data sheet filled out for a child using the program (a blank sheet may be found in the Appendix).

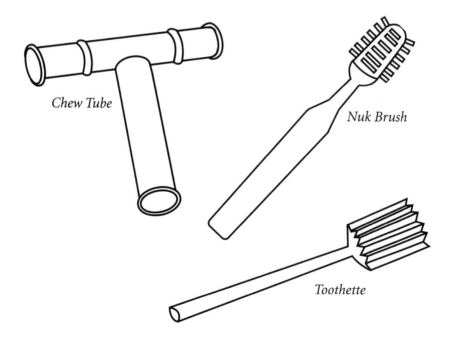

Chew Tube

Nuk Brush

Toothette

	Date 10/7/07 (A) accept (R) reject	Date 10/14/07 (A) accept (R) reject	Date 10/21/07 (A) accept (R) reject
Table 3.2 Sample Oral-Motor Program Data Sheet			
NAME: Amy			
1. Lotion			
a. body:	A	A	A
b. face:	A	A	A
2. ChapStick	A	A	A
3. Nuk brush			
a. lips:	A	A	A
b. tongue			
inside of mouth:	R	(A) 1x (R) 2x	(A) 3x
outside of mouth:	A	A	A
sides of the tongue:	R	(A) on left, (R) on right	(A) on both sides
4. Chew tube	A	A	A
a. consecutive chew:	no	no	no
b. right side:	10 chews, stop and start	10 chews, stop and start	15, stop and start
c. left side:	9 chews, stop and start	15 chews, stop and start	15 stop and start
5. Other	A, mini massager	A, Toothette®	A, flavor spray/Nuk

Some of the other items in the oral-motor box may be presented to the child at this time. Examples include battery-operated toothbrushes, mini massagers, Toothettes®, small foam brushes on a stick, flavored tongue depressors, whistles, hum-a-zoos, finger brushes, flavor sprays, and flavored gloves.

- *Flavor sprays* – may be sprayed on the chew tube, Nuk brush, Toothettes, or finger brush to help the child tolerate them better in the mouth and to increase the amount of oral input. However, not all children enjoy the taste of the flavor spray; it may be too much input at one time. Dipping the Nuk brush or finger brush in water may be a better option for allowing tactile input in their mouths.

- *Small washcloth* – may be dipped in water. Children usually enjoy sucking water off the washcloth. The soft cloth fills their mouths, giving tactile stimulation to the tongue, palate, biting edges of the teeth, gums, and cheeks. This is something that they can be encouraged to chew on, rub their gums with, and use to wipe their mouths.

- *Flavored gloves* – may be worn by the parent, teacher, or therapist. Gloves may be used to rub the child's gums in an organized manner, push on the body of the tongue and the sides of the tongue, rub the inside of the cheeks, and encourage licking movements inside and outside of the mouth.

- *Massagers* – may be used by the child on her face, lips, under the chin, or inside the mouth. It is important that the child is in control of the amount of time that she uses the massager. She is the one who knows when she has had enough stimulation and needs to stop.

- *Whistles, hum-a-zoos, or bubbles* may be demonstrated to the child to encourage him to imitate and join in on the fun.

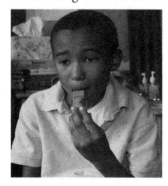

Child using whistle.

By now the child's oral structures have been prepared for improved oral awareness, more normalized oral sensitivity, increased grading and separation of movement, and a more normalized oral feedback system. The oral-motor program performed with the materials in the oral-motor bag should be followed by activities that facilitate oral movements, as outlined in the following.

Activities

This section provides information about food that can be used to promote mature oral movement patterns as well as food that typically facilitates immature and compensatory oral movement patterns and, therefore, should be avoided. Also presented are ideas for activities that encourage movement of the oral structures after being prepared for mature movement patterns through use of the oral-motor program. In addition, the developmental stages of imitation are described to help parents and teachers engage in sound play and speech production with the child.

Foods

In typical development, oral-motor skills, feeding skills, and speech-language skills all develop together and build on each other. The child uses the same muscles for eating as he does for speaking. A meal or snack is a good activity to follow the oral-motor program as eating a variety of foods can further assist in increasing oral stability, mobility, and awareness.

Crunchy solids: Most children enjoy chewing crunchy solids because they provide stimulation. Crunchy solids can facilitate improved chewing skills and jaw stability. Examples include pretzels, carrot sticks, apples, corn chips, potato sticks, toast, crunchy cereals, and rice cakes.

Challenging foods: As the child's chewing skills improve, he can attempt to chew more difficult foods such as lunch meat, chicken nuggets, french fries, dried fruits, and soft cheeses. Other foods such as soft, chewy candy, licorice sticks/twizzlers, fruit roll-ups, marshmallows, and beef jerky can also facilitate chewing skills and jaw stability. Chewing gum may be used to improve jaw stability, facial tone, lip movement, and lateral tongue movement. Finally, cereal, raisins, and chewing gum may be used to encourage side to side movement in the mouth across midline. It is always important to first make sure that the child is capable of chewing these challenging foods.

Foods that encourage sucking: These foods, such as citrus foods, improve tongue and lip control. Citrus foods to try include orange slices/quarters, lemon quarters, lemonade, and lime or orange juice bars. The cold temperature of the juice bars tends to increase oral stimulation, awareness, and sucking movements. Thickened juices, milkshakes, and lollipops can also facilitate sucking. Straws of different shapes and sizes may be used with thickened drinks to increase the amount of sucking needed to drink the liquid.

Foods with a strong taste: This type of food can increase oral awareness and oral sensitivity. This is why children with oral hypo-sensitivity or low tactile awareness often crave spicy foods. Examples include food dips such as salsa and ketchup, sour candies, pickles, and lemons. Cold foods such as ice chips also increase oral awareness.

Foods to Avoid

There are also foods that should NOT be given to children who are having difficulty chewing, sucking, transferring food, and/or swallowing. These include the following.

Nuts and popcorn: These are difficult to chew and should, therefore, be avoided.

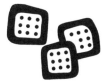

Small pieces of cereal: These may also be problematic because they do not provide the child much sensory feedback about where the cereal is in his mouth.

Foods that stick to the roof of the mouth: An example is a peanut butter and jelly sandwich on soft, white bread. This should be avoided because it facilitates a forward tongue movement when removing it from the top of the mouth or palate. Pieces of the sandwich can also remain on the palate and fall into the mouth later, causing a choking hazard.

A solution would be to toast the bread and cut it into small pieces or strips. The child might also be given a sandwich spread on a cracker broken into smaller pieces. This would facilitate chewing and lateral tongue movement rather than a forward tongue movement. Giving the child small pieces of food would also be helpful if the child typically overstuffs her mouth.

Foods with two or more textures: An example is chicken noodle soup. The child has to swallow the liquid while breaking down the solid pieces of chicken and noodle at the same time. What typically happens is that the solid is swallowed whole with the liquid, which can cause a choking hazard. Thicker soups that have one texture, such as tomato soup, are a good alternative.

Thin liquids should be thickened if the child is gulping the thin liquid with wide jaw excursions. This may be accompanied with the tongue under the cup, which means that tongue movement is not being used for the swallow. This situation might cause the child to aspirate the liquid. The liquid may be thickened with yogurt, applesauce, cornstarch, or commercial products designed to thicken liquids.

A thicker liquid such as nectars may also be used. The thickened drink could be taken through a straw, which would help to slow down the drinking process, facilitate lip closure, and encourage active tongue movement inside of the mouth rather than a forward tongue movement. The straw should be wide enough to allow the child to easily drink the liquid.

Spout cups should not be used with children who have delayed or disordered oral-motor development as they encourage primitive mouth movements. An alternative would be a thermos with a built-in straw or a cup with a top that has a wide lip and holes to allow the liquid to slowly come out.

Oral Movements/Verbalizations

The oral-motor program presented earlier prepared the child's mouth and should be followed by activities that promote movement. This allows for greater success while participating in the planned activities and improved carry-over of the targeted movements into other situations. The child will be better able to integrate the sensations experienced during these activities and produce adaptive responses. This is how sensory integration develops (Ayers, 1979). The oral exercises should be simple and fun.

Blowing activities. Blowing activities facilitate lip closure/control, cheek control, tongue control, jaw control, and controlled inhalation/exhalation.

One example of a blowing activity is blow air hockey. A straw and a cotton ball are used to replace the puck on a tabletop air hockey game. The children can take turns attempting to make their cotton ball go in the goal. Another option is cotton ball races across a table top, blowing the cotton ball with a straw or tube whistle.

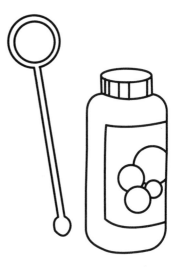

Many children enjoy bubbles. A variety of bubble wands are available that can be tried to assist with the ability to blow bubbles. Blowing can also begin with the child blowing a bubble off a wand by exhaling and saying "ha." This may be demonstrated by saying "ha" on the child's hand and then encouraging her to imitate it. The child can also be encouraged to blow bubbles that are already off the wand.

Candy bubbles are often motivating and helpful if the child tends to suck in the bubbles with the bubble wand rather than blowing out. The child can catch the candy bubbles on her tongue or lips. This facilitates motor planning and oral awareness.

A variety of whistles are available of varying difficulty, sizes, shapes, and sounds. The child can be shown how to make short/long sounds or quiet/loud sounds with the whistles. This works on the child's control of inhalation and exhalation. Hum-a-zoos are especially good, because the child uses his voice to activate them.

Humming. Humming encourages sustained lip closure, phonation, and controlled exhalation.

It is fun for children to hum to music or to just hum a song together. If the child does not hum following encouragement and modeling, model an /a/ sound for him to imitate. Once the child has produced /a/, you can assist with lip closure for humming and encourage the child to sustain this lip closure while continuing to vocalize. If the child does not produce an /a/ sound, gently push on his abdomen after an inhalation of air while modeling the /a/ sound. This should facilitate /a/ or /h/ sounds, which can be shaped into a /m/ sound for humming.

If this is too difficult for the child, encourage him to make any sound or noise. The child can be surrounded by others vocalizing and verbalizing through songs, finger plays, counting, or saying/singing the ABCs. Music CDs that slow down the rate of the songs or songs that have repeated choruses and rhythms are recommended, as they make it easy and fun for you and the child/children to vocalize together. Hand movements and gestures to accompany songs also facilitate the child/children vocalizing with you.

Tongue, lip, and cheek movements. Better tongue movements also improve lip and cheek movements. Working on one tends to assist with improvement of the other; however, all should be addressed during a treatment program.

Sucking small, round lollipops can improve tongue, lip, and cheek movements. Encourage the child to suck the lollipop with lip closure and cheek movement while using the tongue to hold the lollipop against the top of the mouth. You can have a race with the child/children to see who can make the lollipop the smallest the fastest.

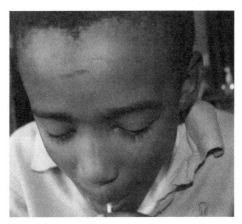

Child closing lips on a lollipop.

Other activities with the lollipop include

- holding the lollipop with lip closure and active cheek movement in the mouth and then pulling the lollipop out of the mouth to make a pop sound

- smacking the lollipop with the lips while holding it in between the lips

- licking the lollipop while it is both inside and outside of the mouth

- rubbing lollipop on the lips and licking it off

- rubbing the lollipop on the tongue to see who can change the color of the tongue the fastest and using the tongue to play hide and seek with the lollipop

These activities are all meant to encourage oral awareness and separate lip and tongue movement from jaw movement. Look for a graded mouth opening and observe the relationship between tongue movement, lip movement, and the size of the mouth opening. For example, the child should be able to move the tongue out of the mouth without a wide mouth opening and move the tongue back into the mouth while maintaining the same open mouth. Often the child closes her mouth when the tongue is brought back into the mouth, indicating that the tongue and the jaw are moving together.

Use jaw control (Redstone, 2004), resting the thumb under the chin and the middle finger under the chin with the non-dominant hand (see page 48), to assist with this if the child needs and accepts it.

This support is light and gives guidance rather than stopping jaw movement. Ice pops can also be presented to the child if she can tolerate the cold temperature. The cold temperature may increase the amount of tongue, lip, and cheek movement due to the increased sensory input.

Pieces of cereal can also be used to assist with improved tongue, lip, and cheek movements. Ask the child to protrude his tongue and hold the cereal on the end of the tongue for a count of 10. As the child gets better at this, ask him to hold the cereal for a higher count. The difficulty of this task may be increased by asking the child to hold the cereal on the tip of the tongue. These tasks promote tongue stability and awareness of the blade and tip of the tongue. While the cereal is still on the tongue, the tongue can then be moved inside to the top of the mouth in an attempt to crush the cereal against the top of the mouth. This facilitates vertical tongue movement and oral awareness. The child can also be asked to move the cereal from side to side inside of the mouth without using head or jaw movements.

From our knowledge of normal development, we know that a child should be able to smoothly move food from side to side inside of the mouth by at least 2 years of age (Evans-Morris & Dunn-Klein, 1987). This indicates that the child has developed jaw stability, separate tongue, cheek, and lip movement, lateral tongue movement, and the ability to plan simple oral movements. The child may also be asked to hold the cereal between her lips for a count of 10 without dropping the cereal. As this becomes easier for the child, it may be increased to a higher count.

Imitation Skills

Imitation is essential for developing speech and language skills (Marshalla, 2001). It teaches the child to participate in turn-taking routines, listen to the speech of others, and also listen to his own sounds or speech production. Children with difficulty registering sensory information, modulating sensory information, organizing and planning simple movements, and initiating movements, as is the case for many on the autism spectrum, do not always develop these skills. These are the symptoms of poor sensory processing that Ayers (1979) described.

After preparing the child's oral system with the oral-motor program as described so far, it is a good time to encourage imitation of oral movements, sounds, words, and phrases. Imitation is a significant part of normal speech and language development where children copy the movements, sounds and words that they see and hear in their everyday environment. Children with ASD would have greater success progressing through the stages of imitation (see Table 3.3) after their oral structures have been prepared for movement.

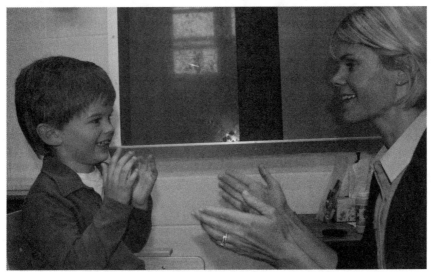

Child and mother playing imitation game.

Table 3.3
Developmental Stages of Imitation

1. **The child vocalizes together with another person.** This may be facilitated by waiting for the child to begin vocalizing and matching the vocalization. Vocalize along with the child and try to sound like him. This helps to draw the child outside of himself and also assists him in listening better to himself and to others. Providing an environment conducive to sound play with singing, music, or gross-motor play can help to initiate vocalizations (Marshalla, 2001).

2. **The child takes turns producing sounds with another.** For example, the child says "m.", the parent, teacher, or therapist says "m, mama" back, and the child then takes his turn and makes another sound. NOTE: Taking turns is what is important here (Marshalla, 2001).

3. **The child learns to imitate himself.** They can be any sounds, such as animal noises, raspberry sounds (a blowing movement with the tongue or lips), oooo's, ahhs, mm, and so on. Any sounds that the child is already making can be part of the imitative sound play (Marshalla, 2001).

   A pause/wait time between imitating what the child has said and him repeating is essential because it is difficult for children with ASD to initiate movements even when the movements are part of their repertoire. Resist the need to fill in this pause time with more speech (Marshalla, 2001).

   This is a good opportunity to add meaning to the child's utterances. For example, the parent, teacher, or therapist could respond with /m/, *more* or /m/, *Mommy* after the child's production of /m/ (Marshalla, 2001).

   You can also imitate movements such as blow, click tongue, and lick lips with the child. These, along with facial expressions, might be produced while sitting in front of a mirror or face-to-face, depending on how the child responds to his mirror image. Again, it is important to imitate the child's production of these movements. The child is only able to imitate himself at this stage of imitation. Therefore, the child must be the one who initiates the sound play, oral movements, or facial expressions.

4. **The child is able to imitate a sound or sound sequence that is already part of his sound repertoire when initiated by someone else.** It is best if these sounds or movements are presented when the child is in the mood to produce them or when the environment is conducive. An example of a conducive mood or environment would be while the child is engaged in movement during a gross-motor activity and already producing sound play (Marshalla, 2001).

   The parent or therapist could initiate with "whee," "go," or whatever sound or verbalization the child has produced in the past, while swinging. A pause would follow, waiting for the child to fill this in with "whee" or "go."

   The oral-motor program will facilitate the child's ability to imitate the movements and sounds in her repertoire when initiated by someone else. Specifically, the first step in the protocol, rubbing with lotion, will help to calm her sensory system so that she can engage in gross-motor play either by herself or with others. The use of the ChapStick, chew tube, and Nuk brush further helps to calm her system. The use of these tools also increases the child's ability to accept touch from her lips and tongue inside and outside of her mouth so that she will want to use these oral structures to imitate and produce sounds.

5. **The child is able to produce novel, single words**. He learns to sequence sounds in a particular way each time and produces a word (Marshalla, 2001). While the child with ASD may be able to produce new, single words spontaneously, it still may be difficult for him to say the word again upon request due to motor planning problems.

   Using routines in which the child has produced a particular word or phrase before might help stimulate the child to produce them again in a novel situation. Examples include songs or books with repeating words or phrases that the child has learned and produced in the past. You are helping him to practice saying words/phrases, rewarding his attempts to spontaneously produce word/phrase productions, and increasing his desire to be verbal.

   The oral-motor program assists with the child's single-word and phrase productions because it establishes a routine where the language remains the same each time. For example, the child is instructed to "take out the Nuk brush." Because this phrase remains relatively the same each time, the child learns to say and practice these words and phrases in an ongoing activity that reinforces comprehension and production of the word or phrase. He then begins to use them on his own to direct others, to question, and to comment.

   Any routine or activity that uses predictable language can be implemented to help the child to master this final stage of imitation where he learns to sequence sounds or words in the same way each time and produce appropriate spontaneous language in a novel situation.

Summary

This chapter provided information on setting up the treatment environment, the treatment program, and activities that can make use of the improved oral system and promote more normalized oral movement patterns. Parents and teachers can easily use the program in the home or at school. Similarly, therapists can use it with the parents and teachers of the children on their caseload. This in turn will support their own treatment programs and assist with carry-over of skills. ■

CHAPTER 4

Incorporating Treatment into Daily Routines

I ncorporating the oral-motor program into the child's daily routine at home and in the classroom will help ensure generalization and consistency. More important, the child's oral-motor, speech, and eating skills will improve if the intervention strategies are implemented on a regular basis.

In this chapter, we will explore ways to make the oral-motor program a habitual part of the classroom and home without adding extra work for parents and teachers. Positions, foods, and activities that support the oral-motor program are also discussed. Finally, case stories of boys with a diagnosis of autism will illustrate how the oral-motor program was easily followed within the classroom setting, even when they were functioning on different levels.

In the Classroom

In the classroom, the oral-motor program – whether conducted within a group setting or individually – can be a regularly scheduled activity. It may be implemented during the child's break time, sensory time, or prior to lunch or snack. This is where the program can most easily be presented to the whole group.

The program may also be used to calm a child who has become over-stimulated due to difficulty processing sensory information occurring at the moment or as a result of an accumulation of sensory input over the course of the day. The program would then be added to the child's schedule as an extra activity. Following is an example of a child's daily morning schedule at school.

Table 4.1 Daily Schedule
1. Putting away backpack and hanging up coat
2. Greeting classmates and teachers
3. Morning group
4. Oral-motor group
5. Language arts
6. Sensory break in OT room
7. Math group
8. Oral-motor: Nuk brush and chew tube
9. Lunch

Each child should have his own oral-motor box in his desk or work area (see Table 3.1). The oral-motor program could be led or monitored by the speech-language pathologist, who would provide feedback and guidance to the teacher about the effect of the oral-motor program on the children's oral-motor, eating, and speech skills. The occupational therapist also plays an important role by offering essential input on how the child is processing sensory information and making recommendations for how to promote acceptance of the oral-motor program within the classroom and home setting. Such suggestions might include activities or routines which can be done with the child during the sensory break in the OT room.

In addition to doing the whole oral-motor program, parts of the program may be integrated into classroom routines by the teacher. For example, a Nuk brush or a battery-operated toothbrush, if the child tolerates more input, and a chew tube, may be used during the regularly scheduled toothbrushing time. Also, following snack or lunch, lotion can be rubbed on the child's face after she washes it, in the manner described in the treatment section.

The use of the Comprehensive Autism Planning System (CAPS) would help to ensure consistency with the oral-motor program throughout the child's day and at home. This system, developed by the professionals and parents, would show the child's use of the oral-motor program over the course of each day and what sensory strategies or supports are needed. There is also a generalization column on the CAPS that would help parents and teachers document other times over the course of the day when they were creatively able to incorporate the oral-motor program or portions of it (Henry & Myles, 2007).

Comprehensive Autism Planning System (CAPS)

Child/Student: _____

*ss=state standard

Time	Activity	Targeted Skills to Teach	Structure/ Modifications	Reinforcement	Sensory Strategies	Communication/ Social Skills	Data Collection	Generalization Plan

Figure 4.1. CAPS.

From Henry, S. A., & Myles, B. S. (2007). *The Comprehensive Autism Planning System (CAPS) for Individuals with Asperger Syndrome, Autism, and Related Disabilities.* Shawnee Mission, KS: Autism Asperger Publishing Company. www.asperger.net; used with permission.

At Home

The oral-motor program can also be part of the routine at home, which will help to ensure generalization and even greater success. It is helpful if the parents can observe the oral-motor program at school so they will better know what to do at home. The program is more likely to be completed on a regular basis if it is part of the home routine. In this way, it will not be forgotten because it is not something extra that needs to be a part of the family's busy day.

The success of the oral-motor program at home and school can be communicated through use of a notebook. This assists with the speech-language pathologist's ability to monitor the child's progress and offer helpful suggestions to the parents and teachers. It can also communicate helpful tips that made the program successful with the child that day at home or school.

Bath Time

The oral-motor program may be incorporated into the child's bath time. Here a soft,
wet washcloth can be used to rub the child's
legs, feet, arms, hands, and face with lotion in
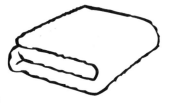
the way that was described in Chapter 3. While the tub is
still filling with water, the child can be given a wet wash cloth, Nuk brush, or chew tube to put in her mouth. Lotion could be rubbed on the child in the manner described in the program after bath time or prior to bed time.

Portions of the program can also be used during the child's nightly tooth-brushing routine. The chew tube and Nuk brush can be added at this time, or the child's regular toothbrush can be used to brush the tongue along with the teeth. (These may also be given to the child while riding in the car or watching television.)

Bed Time

Researchers (Field, 2001) have found that structured tactile input helped to improve sleep patterns, decrease disruptive behaviors, and increase the ability of children with autism to relate to others.

The oral-motor program provides structured tactile input that can help to calm the child in preparation for sleep in addition to improving oral-motor skills. This would also assist with other bedtime routines such as verbal imitation of words or phrases while reading books, singing songs, or other night time rituals.

Oral-Motor Box/Bag

An oral-motor box (see Table 3.1) should be made for the child to have available at home. It may be given to the child prior to meal time as a routine part of the family's daily schedule. The box or bag may be kept in the kitchen and used as part of the child's preparation for the meal.

If the oral-motor program has been used with the child on a daily basis, he should be able to be independent with the components in the oral-motor box/bag. The parents can just ask the child to get the oral-motor box and he will be able to use the different items on his own in the manner that has been used in the past.

Other Activities That Support Treatment

When parents and teachers understand why it is important to work on a particular skill with the child, it is easier for them to see different opportunities to support it over the course of the day. This section gives suggestions for how to accomplish this, including stable positioning, food, singing, using a microphone, and playing.

Positioning

One of the best ways to support treatment throughout the day is by proper positioning. As mentioned, the child's oral structures move best if the child is in a stable position with her body in midline, the head/neck in a flexed position, and the feet touching the floor (Redstone, 2004). This body posture should be used as much as possible throughout the day; for example, at the dining table, during fine-motor activities, and while watching television, reading, and/or during speech production. It is important that the child is at eye level while watching television, reading, during classroom activities, or social interactions. This discourages hyper-extending the head and neck, excessive fixing of the musculature at the head, neck, and shoulders, and a locked forward or backward posture of the jaw, tongue, and lips, all of which inhibit movement for speech production or eating.

As mentioned, beanbag chairs are appropriate for some activities as they can be shaped to provide the correct body posture for the child. Children often enjoy these chairs because they surround them and give tactile input about where they are in space. If additional tactile input is needed or enjoyed by the child, a second beanbag chair can be placed on the child's lap, or a weighted blanket may be used.

Food That Encourages Mature Oral Patterns

Another way to support treatment throughout the day is by offering the child food types that encourage mature oral patterns, such as crunchy solids that encourage chewing movements to develop jaw stability. By practicing the mature oral patterns during eating, these patterns will be more available during speech production. These food types, described in the Foods section in Chapter 3, can assist with increased oral awareness, the development of jaw stability, increased lip, cheek, and tongue movements, and the development of separate movement of the tongue and lips from the jaw.

As foods are incorporated throughout the day, it is important to pay careful attention to the foods to be avoided or to be presented in a different manner for the child who is producing immature or atypical oral movements (see Chapter 3). For example, a thin semi-solid like yogurt might encourage a forward-backward tongue movement when taken from a spoon. This is an immature, primitive oral movement pattern, seen in Table 2.1 in the birth to 3 months section. If the child is practicing this pattern while eating, it is likely that he is also using this pattern during speech production. An alternative would be to have him drink the yogurt through a straw. This facilitates lip closure and the tongue being pulled back into the mouth, which are important movements in preparation for speech.

Singing

Singing is a great way to encourage oral movements, sound production, and prosody or rhythm. Speech becomes slower, more rhythmical, and continuous when you sing. Many children with ASD have difficulty starting and stopping their production of sound. With singing, the speech sound becomes prolonged and continuous, making it easier for the child to maintain and initiate phonation or the production of sound.

Songs with repeated choruses or hand movements are especially helpful and fun, but any song will work. Ask the child to sing along and make sounds just for fun. The child's ability to vocalize along with the music is more important than him being able sing all the words to the song.

Microphones

Microphones often motivate children to produce sound and are a great way to encourage them to listen to themselves. The amplification from the microphone will help to focus and sustain the child's attention on the task of producing sounds. As with singing, the child should be encouraged to vocalize and have fun.

Play

On the playground, the child may be encouraged to vocalize sounds and/ or words repeatedly such as "ooh," "wheee," "yea" while playing on the equipment. This makes sound play fun and easy. These types of sounds can also be used to engage other children on the playground since they are vocalizations/words produced by many children while moving about on a playground.

Assign meaning to any of the child's vocalizations that are produced consistently over a period of time. This will encourage the child to continue production of the sound sequence and help him to use it in an appropriate context.

Case Stories

The following case stories describe three boys, all of whom have a diagnosis of autism and attend a school for children with autism. (A case study involving a student in a public school may be found in Chapter 5.) The boys are very different, but each benefited from the oral-motor program. The program was considered successful for each of them for different reasons and was continued on a regular basis, as illustrated in the following.

Michael

Michael, an 8-year-old boy with a diagnosis of
autism, infrequently produced sounds but was
able to make the vowel sounds /u/ as in *cup*,
/a/ as in *mop*, /ae/ as in *hat* and /e/ sound as in
me. Michael had a voice output device with a
dynamic screen. He did not use this device to
spontaneously initiate communication but used
it when verbally or physically prompted by an adult. He imitated the signs
more, finished, help, me, bathroom, eat, and *drink* but did not use them spontaneously to initiate communication. If he did not like an activity or object,
he communicated this by yelling or crying.

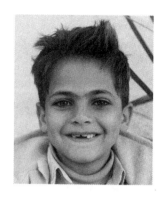

Michael ate different food types but chewed his food in rapid, small bites
without variety in the range of movements of the lower jaw. In typical
development, this type of movement would be called munching. It is an
example of a delayed movement pattern, whereby food is mashed against
the palate and the biting edges of the teeth in preparation for a swallow.
It is seen in the normally developing population at approximately 5 to 6
months of age, when babies are first exposed to semi-solids with a lumpy
texture (Evans-Morris & Dunn-Klein, 1987). Smooth semi-solids were
taken from a spoon by scraping the food off with the upper teeth and
swallowing with minimal lip movement and forward/backward tongue
movement. Michael held the cup back in his mouth while biting on the
cup edge. He drank one sip at a time with an audible gulp.

Michael refused a Nuk brush or chew tube when held in front of his
mouth by an adult facing him. He did this by yelling and pushing away
with his hand. He would gag if an adult attempted to touch his lips with
a gloved hand. His tongue, cheeks, and lips were held tightly in a pulled-
back position. The muscles that formed the base of the tongue were also
held in a fixed, tight position.

Michael did not imitate simple oral movements such as "stick out your tongue," "lick your lips," "hum," or "click your tongue." He did blow upon request. He was unable to imitate individual speech sounds, including the vowel sounds that were part of his verbal repertoire. He often became agitated when asked to imitate oral movements or speech sounds.

Oral-motor group. Oral-motor group using the program presented in earlier chapters was started in Michael's classroom by the speech-language pathologist. Each child sat with his or her teaching assistant around a table. Michael was given an oral-motor bag that included a Nuk brush, chew tube, whistles, hum-a-zoo, mini massager, flavored lip balm (e.g., ChapStick), Toothettes, and lotion.

The session began by asking the children to take off their shoes and socks. They were then instructed to rub lotion on one leg and foot, the other leg and foot; one arm and hand, then the other arm and hand, and finally, the face. Michael tolerated only a small amount of lotion, which he rubbed in by himself. His teaching assistant encouraged him to continue to rub in the lotion on each body part while the group sang a song about the activity and various body parts.

After lotion, the mini massager was handed to Michael. He enjoyed the vibration on the bottoms of his feet, the palms of his hands, behind his ear, on his cheeks and lips, and under his chin. It was important that Michael provide this stimulation to himself because, due to his poor tactile awareness, he rejected tactile input from others and became tactically defensive and aggressive (Ayers, 1979; Yack et al., 2002). When he held the massager, he enjoyed it for a relatively long period of time. He put the massager down when he had enough of it.

Michael was then instructed to take out his lip balm. He easily put the flavored lip balm on his lips, because this was an activity that he was familiar with in order to protect his lips in the winter time. The lotion, lip balm, and the mini massager helped to prepare Michael's body to tolerate tactile input inside of the mouth where he was very sensitive and defensive.

He was next asked to take out his chew tube, put it in his mouth, and chew. He held it at his lips while the group counted and clapped to a specified number. He was encouraged but never forced to put the chew tube in his mouth.

The children were then instructed to "put away your chew tubes and take out your Nuk brush." (The chew tube was cleaned with an alcohol wipe or alcohol spray prior to being put back in the oral-motor bag. The same was true for the Nuk brush.) Michael held his own Nuk brush and was encouraged to push down on his tongue inside of his mouth with the brush while the adults counted and clapped a specified number of times. The children were also encouraged to push on the sides of their tongue and brush the top of their mouth. Michael held the Nuk brush and opened his mouth. With prompting, he was able to touch the tip of his tongue, without gagging. This was applauded and seen as success.

The children were next instructed to put away their Nuk brushes and take out a whistle or hum-a-zoo. Michael was able to blow, so this was an easy activity for him. He had a variety of whistles in his oral-motor bag that he insisted on blowing once or twice before putting them back in his bag.

An activity that encouraged use of the oral structures followed this routine. This was either based on something in the classroom curriculum or on an oral movement that needed to be worked on with the group. For example, if the class curriculum was emphasizing clothing worn in the winter, a story about winter would be read to the group, and the sounds of winter would be emphasized such as the wind went "ooooooh." The group was then encouraged to join in with the sound play.

During the initial oral-motor groups, games that included blowing (see Chapter 3) were often presented since this was a successful activity for Michael. An example would be blowing a cotton ball with a straw back and forth between two children. The students also used a small air hockey game and blew cotton balls with a straw across the table to make a goal.

Oral-motor group continued with the class on a weekly basis for a 30-minute block of time. The speech-language pathologist led the group with the specific language for each item in the oral-motor bag. The children and/or the teaching assistants performed the actions with each item during group time. The speech-language pathologist moved from child to child to ensure the child and/or teaching assistant did each exercise properly. She also completed the oral-motor data sheet (see page 51) at this time. Lotion, the chew tube, and the Nuk brush were also on Michael's daily classroom schedule.

Michael did the oral-motor program under the supervision of his teaching assistant, who had been individually trained by the speech-language pathologist on how to use the items in the oral-motor bag and was also part of the weekly oral-motor group.

Table 4.2 Michael's Oral-Motor Program	
Major Deficits	*Treatment Protocol*
Tactile defensiveness	• Rub lotion himself on his feet, legs, arms, hands, and face • Use mini massager himself on feet, legs, arms, hands, face, tongue • Apply lip balm himself to his lips
Hypersensitive to touch	• Use chew tube and Nuk brush himself, prompted with verbal and nonverbal instructions
Poor jaw stability	• Prompt to chew 10 to 30 times on each side with the chew tube
Poor use of cheeks/lips	• Use whistles and blowing games

Results of oral-motor group. Michael's oral-motor skills began to change after initiation of this intensive oral-motor program. After six months, he tolerated all the items in his oral-motor bag both outside and inside of his mouth. His teaching assistant was able to help him rub lotion on himself, guide his chew tube onto his teeth edges, and help him brush the top of his mouth and the body, sides, and tip of his tongue with his Nuk brush. He no longer gagged when someone other than himself touched his mouth. He was able to imitate the /m,b,d,n/ sounds in consonant-vowel words with the vowel sounds that were part of his repertoire. He produced the words *no* and *all done* spontaneously to reject objects and events. His cheeks, lips, and tongue continued to be retracted but with less severity. His chewing pattern was replaced with varied, vertical jaw movements, which was a more mature pattern (Evans-Morris & Dunn-Klein, 1987). Downward, upper-lip movement was used to clean the spoon. While drinking from a cup, he continued to bite on the cup edge and take one sip at a time. He no longer produced the audible gulps after thickened liquids were recommended for him at school and at home. Michael was able to produce a tongue click, lick his lips, and stick his tongue out when given a visual and verbal model.

Currently, Michael is 11 years old. He continues to participate in oral-motor group once a week for 30 minutes, and the oral-motor program is still part of his daily schedule with his teaching assistant. Michael participates actively and independently completes all the activities in oral-motor group. He gets his oral-motor bag by himself and sits at the table when he is told it is time for oral-motor group. He independently follows the one- and two-step directions that are part of the oral-motor group, such as "Put away your chew tube and get out your Nuk brush." Michael often leads the group by singing the song about what he and the rest of the students are doing while rubbing in his lotion. He also leads the group in counting while chewing on his chew tube. For a child who had no verbal language at age 8, this is a significant improvement.

In addition, the activity that follows the oral-motor program is at a higher level than when Michael was 8 years old. For example, the group is now encouraged to produce particular speech sounds within the context of a word. These words are emphasized in a story or activity that is based on classroom curriculum. For example, before and after the students went to a day camp, a book about camp was read to them.

Michael's verbal language has increased significantly since he was 8 years old. He now produces three-, four-, and five-word sentences, and he frequently uses the phrases "I want _____" to request a variety of objects and activities, as well as "no thank you," "yes, please," "I need help," and "I'm all done." He names actions in pictures by producing agent + action + ing + object sentence types. He responds accurately to yes/no, what-doing, and what-question types. He continues to have difficulty initiating language with others. He spontaneously uses his language to reject, answer questions, complete sentences about an object or picture, and participate in routine books, songs, or games.

Anthony

Anthony, a 9-year-old boy with a diagnosis of autism, produced a variety of speech sounds in his spontaneous speech, which contained mostly one-word phrases. His single-word productions were difficult to understand if the topic was not known to the listener. Upon request, Anthony could produce a range of com-

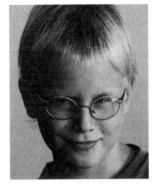

mon oral movements and imitated two- and three-movement sequences of these.

Anthony ate a variety of food types. He did not have any significant problems with his eating skills. He tolerated lotion, a Nuk brush, a chew tube, and a mini massager when presented to him or by him.

Anthony became overstimulated quickly and easily by other people in the room, especially when they were in close proximity. He would show this by flapping his hands, jumping on his toes, producing high-pitched sounds, and pinching himself and others.

Oral-motor group. Oral-motor group was begun in Anthony's classroom by a speech-language pathologist. The students sat around a table with their teaching assistant. Each student had an oral-motor bag that contained lotion, a chew tube, a Nuk brush, a mini massager, a variety of whistles, a lip balm, hum-a-zoos, bubbles, Toothettes, and flavor spray. The speech-language pathologist led the group in the order and with the exact language discussed in Chapter 3. The teaching assistant observed, assisted, or performed the exercises with the child. The speech-language pathologist observed each child to make sure the exercises were done properly and to fill out the oral-motor data sheet.

First the students were instructed to take off their shoes and socks and get out their lotion. Anthony was able to follow this two-step instruction but had difficulty sitting at the table in close proximity to the other students. As a result, he began to produce high-pitched squeals and pinched others around him.

After the initial group, a beanbag chair, placed close to the table, was provided for Anthony to sit in during the oral-motor routine. He was now able to calmly participate in the group activity with his teaching assistant at his side. The sequence of the group followed the same routine as the one described for Michael. Anthony enjoyed rubbing lotion on himself but had difficulty following along with the specific body part being sung about. He liked the mini massager on the bottoms of his feet, on his face, and behind his ear. Anthony was also compliant with applying the lip balm to his lips and easily followed the instruction to get out his chew tube. Chewing on his chew tube in a rhythmical manner a set number of times seemed to calm him. The firm, downward pressure on his tongue with the Nuk brush, also in a rhythmical manner, a set number of times calmed him. After this, the whistles, hum-a-zoo, or bubbles were used by Anthony and the other students in the group.

Table 4.3
Anthony's Oral-Motor Program

Major Deficits	Treatment Protocol
Easily overstimulated by sensory input	• Rub lotion on himself while in a beanbag chair to help calm himself. Apply lip balm to lips, chew 10 to 30 times on the chew tube, firm pressure downward on the body of the tongue 10 to 30 times while inside the mouth with the Nuk brush
Poor awareness of his body	• Sing or name body parts while rubbing lotion on himself. Name parts of the body to which he is applying lip balm, chew tube, Nuk brush, and mini massager
Inability to sequence words	• Use predictable language that is repeated the same way each time during the oral-motor program

Results of oral-motor group. After completing the oral-motor program, Anthony was calmed enough so that he was able to participate in activities at the table with the other students. The activities supported the classroom curriculum or emphasized particular oral movements or speech sounds. One of the activities was a game where the students had to imitate a facial expression pictured on a card and then match the card to a game board containing facial expressions.

The oral-motor program became part of Anthony's daily routine. It was placed on his daily schedule and carried out with his teaching assistant. The chew tube and Nuk brush were presented to him during the day when he became overstimulated and needed assistance to calm himself.

Presently, Anthony is 12 years old. He is able to tolerate sitting at the table for the entire oral-motor group. He knows the routine so well that he can lead the group and give the other students instructions to follow. For example, he will say, "It is time for lotion" or "Get out your chew tube." He is also now able to rub lotion on the body part that is named in the song.

The oral-motor program continues to be part of his daily school schedule. He is able to produce one-, two-, and three-word sentences that are easily understood even if the topic of conversation is not known to the listener. Some of his four-, five-, and six- word phrases can be difficult to understand when the topic of conversation is not known, however. Anthony uses verbal language to spontaneously request and reject objects and events. The Nuk brush and chew tube are presented to him if he is having difficulty calming himself.

George

George, a 13-year-old boy with a diagnosis of autism, produced vowel sounds, such as /o/ in *hot* and /a/ in *hat*, with the g, b, and m consonant sounds while jumping or walking. These sounds were not produced with communicative intent. If he was attending to an adult while producing the sounds, George continued his sound production in a reciprocal manner with the adult. He constantly drooled and frequently had his hands in his mouth. A gag reflex was stimulated on the back of his tongue and on his soft palate.

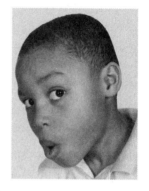

George independently ate a variety of foods, using his hands to place large amounts in his mouth. He stored food in both cheeks that often remained there after he was finished eating his meal. With assistance, he used a spoon or fork to scoop or stab his food; however, he also attempted to grab the food with his hands. He drank from a cup with his tongue under the cup edge but also drank from a small straw placed in a drink box. He swallowed with a forward/backward tongue movement. George used Picture Communication Symbols (PCS) (Mayer-Johnson, 1994-2005) to request a drink versus something to eat. He would hand the PCS with eye contact to an adult. His ability to chose the drink versus the eat symbol was tied to the placement of the two symbols. The PCS and sign language for *wait, more, finish, help, trampoline/jump* and *music* were also used with George.

Oral-motor group. Oral-motor group was initiated in George's classroom and led by a speech-language pathologist. The sequence of the oral-motor program for this group was the same as that described for Michael and Anthony, and the group was led in the same manner as described in the previous case stories. The teaching assistant performed the oral exercises with George. The speech-language pathologist observed the manner in which the oral exercises were performed with George and filled out the oral-motor data sheet. George was given an oral-motor bag that contained a Nuk brush, battery-operated toothbrush, chew tube, mini massager, ChapStick, bubbles, and flavor sprays. George had difficulty sitting in a chair throughout the day. He preferred to stand and jump in place.

For his first oral-motor group, George sat in a beanbag chair with his teaching assistant and the speech-language pathologist on either side of him. His shoes and socks were removed, and his feet, legs, arms, hands, and face were rubbed with lotion while a song was sung to him with the rest of the group. George enjoyed the lotion, mini massager, and the singing and easily remained in the beanbag chair. The chew tube and Nuk brush were presented to him once or twice each. George was then finished and got up from the beanbag chair.

Table 4.4
George's Oral-Motor Program

Major Deficits	Treatment Protocol
Hypo-sensitive to touch	• Rub lotion on feet, legs, arms, hands, face by self or others using firm touch to increase awareness.
Excessive drooling	• Put powder on chin to emphasize feeling of a dry chin. Use lip balm with lip closure to encourage this for swallowing saliva.
Constant fingers in mouth; stuffing large amounts of food in mouth	• Push firmly on the body of the tongue 10 to 30 times with the Nuk brush, brush the sides of the tongue with the Nuk brush, encouraging movement to the side teeth. Also use the Nuk brush to brush the tip of the tongue and the top of the mouth. Use chew tube 10 to 30 times on transitions to discourage fingers in mouth.
Forward/backward tongue movement during the swallow	• Push downward on the body of the tongue with the Nuk brush and then move the Nuk brush to the top of the mouth encouraging the tongue to move vertically rather than forward/backward. • Apply resistance when asking the child to produce this vertical movement.

Results of oral-motor group. George attended oral-motor group every week. Extending the amount of time that he spent in the beanbag chair each week, by the end of the first month, he was sitting in it for the entire oral-motor program. He also sat for the activity that followed if it had anything to do with music. He used his chew tube and Nuk brush the same number of times as the other students in the group. George was not able to follow any of the directions with oral-motor group but accepted the tactile and oral input provided to him by his teaching assistant. This was considered a huge success for him.

The oral-motor program became part of George's daily routine. A PCS for oral-motor was placed on his daily schedule and also became part of his daily routine. He continued to attend the weekly oral-motor group with his teaching assistant. George's drooling decreased following the initiation of the oral-motor group, but his need to keep his fingers in his mouth remained. A chew tube was given to him throughout the day in an attempt to keep his hands out of his mouth.

George is about to turn 14. He now sits at the table in a chair with the other students during oral-motor group with his teaching assistant to assist him. He no longer needs the beanbag chair. He enjoys the oral-motor program during group time and during his daily individual time. George will remain in his chair if the activity following the oral-motor program involves singing or music. If not, he often gets up from his chair with his teaching assistant.

George continues to jump or walk about the room when he is not seated at his desk or at the group table. He will sit in a chair the longest during group and individual oral-motor time. His sound production is still associated with movement. When engaged by an adult, he continues his sound production in a reciprocal manner. The chew tube is given to George throughout the day in order to keep his hands out of his mouth.

George continues to need assistance to eat with a spoon or fork. If given the opportunity, he will grab food with his hands; however, the amount of food he places in his mouth is much less than before, and he no longer stores food in his cheeks. His gag reflex now is produced slightly more forward in the mouth and on the palate. George uses a straw to drink from a cup to avoid tongue placement under the cup and from a box drink. He also drinks thickened liquids to decrease the use of a forward/backward tongue movement during the swallow.

Summary

The suggestions for incorporating the oral-motor program into home and classroom routines presented here will assist with the child's ability to generalize oral skills from the therapy session, thereby improving eating skills and expanding speech/language skills to a variety of situations and events. It will also help to ensure consistency with the child's skills. The case stories allow readers to see how the oral-motor program was used with three boys who had a diagnosis of autism. Each boy had different reasons for using the program, but each benefited tremendously from it. ■

X

CHAPTER 5

Complementary Therapies

Numerous therapy techniques are recommended for children with autism spectrum disorder (ASD), which can be confusing and overwhelming to both parents and professionals. Discussed in this chapter will be therapies that may be used along with the oral-motor program presented in Chapters 3 and 4 to further support the development and improvement of oral-motor, eating, and speech communication skills. The author has received extensive training in neurodevelopmental treatment approach (NDT) and craniosacral therapy. She has completed the Touch for Health courses I through IV, is a certified Bowen practitioner, and has taken the first course in Brain Gym and in the PROMPT technique to be discussed here.

Some of the therapies may work better with one child than with another for individual reasons or may work better with the same child for a certain period of time than another. For this reason, it is helpful to have knowledge of a variety of therapy techniques, such as NDT, craniosacral therapy, the Bowen Technique, Touch for Health, and Brain Gym. These techniques may be described as manipulative and body-based practices, which fall under the category of complementary and alternative medicine. They focus on the structures and systems of the body.

The majority of the research on manipulative and body-based practices has been clinical, such as case studies. There are challenges with performing research with these therapies due to difficulty with the reproduction of the intervention procedures with different practitioners, identification of control groups, and the development of standardized outcome measures (Manipulative and body-based, 2007). This is why there might be a lack of research to support the successes observed during the therapy session.

The technique that works best for the child should be used consistently over a period of time. *Consistency* and *over a period of time* are key terms, especially when working with children with ASD. Because many therapies are touted as the "answer," it is tempting to try different ones without giving any one therapy a chance to succeed. Some families use one type of therapy with the child for a short period of time until another becomes popular. The new therapy is then either added to the current treatment program or implemented exclusively. This pattern of using treatments for short periods of time or randomly adding treatments makes it difficult to ascertain which therapy works best for the child.

The speech-language therapist, the child's parents, and the teachers, as appropriate, should implement a therapy technique for a series of consecutive sessions before making a judgment on whether it should be pursued. "This is where collecting data comes in. Based on what is discovered in the data, interventions may be altered or may be continued as is" (Henry & Myles, 2007, p. 101).

Procedures for Collecting Data

Observational data recording systems allow for observation and recording of behavior as it occurs in the classroom and are particularly useful in analyzing questions such as those that address student response to instruction, student engagement, and student behaviors. Many other systems are also available, as illustrated in Table 5.1.

Table 5.1 **Commonly Used Observational Data Recording Systems**

■ **Event Recording** – an exact measure of behavior
  ◆ use for discrete behaviors (those that have a definite beginning and end)
  ◆ count/tally how many times behavior occurs
    – Examples: raise hand, call out, ask question

■ **Latency Recording** – an exact measure of behavior
  ◆ measure how long it takes to begin something
    – Examples: follow directions, begin work

■ **Duration Recording** – an exact measure of behavior
  ◆ measure how long a behavior persists
    – Examples: temper tantrum, out of seat

■ **Time Sampling** – an estimate of behaviors
  ◆ use for ongoing or high-frequency behaviors
  ◆ record whether behavior is or is not occurring at the end of every specific period of time (for example, every 30 seconds) for a specific session (for example, a session of 5 minutes at the beginning of class)
    – Examples: talk to peers (if high frequency), stay on task

Neurodevelopmental Treatment Approach (NDT)

The Neurodevelopmental Treatment Approach (NDT) was developed in the 1940s by Dr. and Mrs. Bobath to treat individuals with disorders of the central nervous system that resulted in difficulty controlling movement. NDT initially emphasized reflex integration and normal development. It has evolved into an integrated approach that assesses the child's movements to determine which components of movement are interfering with the child's development and function (Redstone, 2007). "It is a theory-driven approach, which is supported by current theories of motor development" (Redstone, 2007, p. 127). It has benefited individuals with mild to severe motor problems.

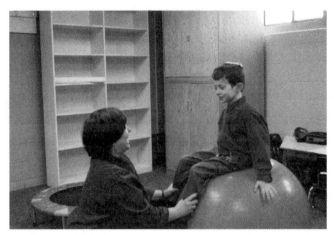

NDT approach.

It has been challenging for NDT-trained therapists to document changes and show that their treatment has been effective with their clients. Clinical trials are not used because withholding treatment is not an option. Also, the flexible way in which NDT principles are practiced and integrated makes it difficult to document and compare outcomes. The evidence to date on the advantages of NDT-based intervention is inconsistent and shows that more research is needed.

The Neurodevelopmental Treatment Association (NDTA) has taken steps to assist with the development of evidence-based practice. Thus, a committee has been established to review the scientific literature, and financial support is available for studies examining the effects of NDT techniques. The NDTA also supports eight-week, advanced training courses for physical therapists, occupational therapists, and speech-language pathologists. This is an attempt to make sure that there is a consistent knowledge base among therapists practicing this method (Howle, 2002).

"An NDT SLP [speech-language pathologist] addresses the motor impairment (abnormal muscle tone, lack of head control, jaw instability) while targeting discipline-specific objectives (lip closure, cause/effect, vocalization) through functional activities (e.g., eating, playing, speech) in an age-appropriate context" (Redstone, 2007, p. 122).

As mentioned in Chapters 1 and 2, children with a diagnosis of ASD often exhibit low muscle tone, leading to a poor base of support, thus affecting all aspects of the child's development. This can cause the child with ASD to "fix" or hold one part of the body in order to move another part of the body. The low muscle tone interferes with stability, mobility, and leads to asymmetry and compensatory movement patterns. An example would be the child who asymmetrically clenches the lower jaw for stability in order to move the tongue and lips for eating or speech production. Such a compensatory pattern inhibits the development of mature oral movements.

The therapist who is NDT-trained would be able to observe the compensatory pattern caused by the low muscle tone and the poor stability and understand how it impacts the whole child. He or she would then devise a treatment program to facilitate mature, normal movement patterns while inhibiting the compensatory patterns that are not part of normal development.

The treatment program would begin with proper positioning so the child would have an adequate base of support. (The child would be sitting with the hips, knees, and feet at a 90-degree angle and the head in midline with a slight chin tuck.) The child's oral ability will improve following proper alignment of the head and trunk (Redstone, 2004). Jaw support or oral control is then used to give the child external support so that he does not need to clench the jaw. This oral control can be provided while sitting in front of the child and using the non-dominant hand. The thumb is placed on the chin and the middle finger is rested under the chin (Redstone, 2004) (see page 48). The support may be used during eating and speech production, guiding the size of the child's mouth opening.

This is how positioning and therapeutic handling are used to help the child develop a functional skill by inhibiting and facilitating movement. The jaw clenching and asymmetrical movements would be inhibited and midline, oral alignment, and graded movements would be facilitated (Redstone, 2007). Parents can find a therapist who is trained in the NDT by contacting the Neurodevelopmental Treatment Association, which is listed in the resource section of the Appendix.

Craniosacral Therapy

John E. Upledger, an osteopathic physician, developed craniosacral therapy in the 1970s and 1980s while at Michigan State University. Soft touch is used in craniosacral therapy to assist with the release of restrictions in the craniosacral system (Hughes, 2004). The cranialsacral system consists of a waterproof container that begins inside the skull vault and extends downward within the vertebral column to the sacralcoccygeal complex or the sacrum and coccyx. It involves all the fluid and membranes that surround the brain and the spinal cord. The fluid inside the cranialsacral system is called cerebrospinal fluid. The cranialsacral system moves in response to the build-up and absorption of the cerebral spinal fluid. This creates a cranial rhythm, and every part of the cranialsacral system moves in response to this rhythm (Hughes, 2004).

The cranialsacral system is interrelated with the fascia system. Fascia is tough connective tissue that is a continuous sheet extending vertically from the top of the head to the tip of the toes. It supports and stabilizes the body. Restrictions in

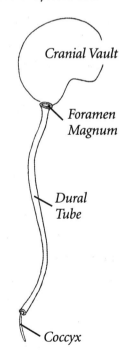

Cranial Vault

Foramen Magnum

Dural Tube

Coccyx

Cranial-Sacral System.

the fascia system can cause a torque anywhere in the cranialsacral system, inhibiting balanced, symmetrical movements.

Craniosacral therapy can mobilize restrictions in the fascia and cranialsacral system, facilitate the body to return to a state of symmetry, and decrease compensatory movement patterns through light touch (Upledger, 2001). The therapist trained in craniosacral therapy learns to listen to the patient's body and, through this light touch, assists him in returning to a state of balance and symmetry.

In his presentation *Autism-Observations, Experiences and Concepts*, Dr. John E. Upledger (Government Reform Committee of the U.S. House of Representatives, 2000) described his etiologic model for autism. According to Upledger, in children with a diagnosis of autism, the "meningeal membranes that line the cranial vault and cover the surface of the brain lose their accommodative growth abilities, thereby disrupting the normal expansion of brain and cranial vault." "The manual stretching of the restrictive dura mater by the use of craniosacral therapy techniques has provided impressive improvement in autism" (Government Reform Committee of the U.S. House of Representatives, 2000). Craniosacral therapy has also been effective in the treatment of children with attention deficit disorder (Upledger, 2001).

The Bowen Technique

The soft tissue manipulation technique was started in Australia by Tom Bowen in the 1950s and is now practiced in more than 30 countries around the world. It is a minimalist approach, based on the philosophy that too much stimulus interferes with the brain's ability to respond (Bowtech, 2006). In other words, with too much stimulus, the brain does not know where to focus its attention. The Bowen Technique helps the body return to a state of equilibrium and balance so that optimal functioning is possible. As such, it releases the restrictions in the body that deplete energy, cause stress, and inhibit movement and organ function.

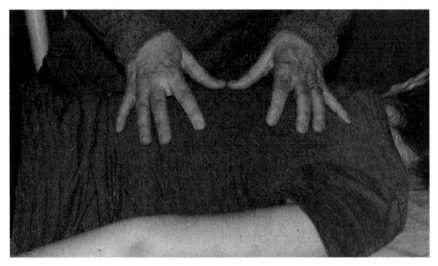

The Bowen Technique.

The Bowen Technique involves a series of precise moves on specific
points of the body, generally over a muscle, tendon, or nerve sheath.
These moves are done with the fingers or thumbs through clothing. First,
the proprioceptors are activated, which then signal the autonomic nervous system. The body's response to the moves resets the tension in the
muscles and other tissues, including a release of the surrounding fascia.
There are frequent pauses between the moves, which gives the body time
to respond and, in turn, gives the child a better sense of his position and
movement through space.

According to Augustyniak (2005), "the genius of Bowen is in the waits"
[between the moves] (p. 8). After a Bowen session, it is recommended
that patients wait 5 to 10 days before the next session, and that they
drink water, walk or otherwise move around (Bowtech, 2006) because
movement helps to integrate the body's responses to the stimulation
provided during the session. "A Bowen treatment also continues healing
and changing the body for 3-5 days after the treatment as though the
person received a treatment everyday" (Augustyniak, 2005, p. 10).

As mentioned earlier, children with a diagnosis of ASD are often in an alert state of "flight or fight," which originates in the sympathetic portion of the autonomic nervous system. These series of precise moves over a particular muscle and nerve sheath send signals via the proprioceptors to the brain through the autonomic nervous system and help the child to relax. This assists with balancing the sympathetic portion of our nervous system so the child will not remain in "flight or fight."

Effects of Bowen Technique

Parents have reported to this author that their child, with a diagnosis of ASD, is calmer and more attentive after a Bowen session. Similarly, a case control study by Whitaker, Gilliam, and Seba (1997) concluded that the autonomic nervous system was affected by the Bowen Technique. The group treated with the Bowen Technique showed heart rate variability, which is controlled by the autonomic nervous system, and symptom relief perception.

Sandra Gustafson, ND, RN, and senior instructor of the Bowen Therapy Academy of Australia, stated in her article "Maternal & Newborn Care" (2007) that the Bowen Technique has successfully been used to treat babies with feeding difficulties, colic, and reflux. She notes, "It is completely safe, is not known to have any undesired side effects, and can be used in nearly every health condition to improve the quality of people's lives" (Gustafson, 2007, p. 3).

Further, a Bowen practitioner in New Zealand reported on a 4-1/2-year-old boy who, during the first session, spoke in single, one-syllable words that were difficult to understand, and was not walking or crawling. After the 15th session, this boy's speech was described as "clear," and he was pulling himself up to stand (Richardson, 2004).

Touch for Health

Dr. Thie developed Touch for Health to make available some of the basic principles of applied kinesiology, a method for studying human movement, to the general public. It is based on a triangle of health, which looks at a person's mental/emotional, structural, and biochemical dimensions. When these dimensions are in balance, the person is said to exist in a state of health.

Touch for Health teaches how to balance these dimensions. It also tests for muscle imbalances through muscle testing or monitoring. Information gained allows the therapist trained in this technique to balance a weak muscle with an over-energized muscle so that there can be harmony between the two opposing muscles. In other words, if a muscle is tight, it is because the opposing muscle is weak or not working against it (Touch for Health, 1973).

The Touch for Health (1973) treatment protocol allows the therapist trained in this technique to assess the areas of imbalance, indicate patterns of need, and show where the focus of treatment should be in the body. Correcting for these imbalances allows the muscles to relax and facilitates movement by allowing the structure to normalize, ultimately, helping the body to function more efficiently with less stress. Touch for Health (1973) techniques balance the whole system.

In children with ASD, the emotional stress release (ESR) technique can be used to help decrease the "fight or flight" reflex. This is done by gently holding the child's forehead (Touch for Health, 1973).

Brain Gym

Brain Gym, developed by Paul E. Dennison and Gail E. Dennison, consists of a series of movements and activities that enhance the ability to learn with the whole brain. Specifically, the movements and activities stimulate organization, release the inability to focus, and facilitate relaxation so information can be processed without fear, or a "fight-or-flight" response. Thus, Brain Gym frees the child for learning to take place and enhances automatic, whole-body learning (Brain Gym, 1998).

Effects of Brain Gym

Carla Hannaford (1995) examined the effects of Brain Gym with a group of 19 fifth-grade special education students. The Brigance Inventory of Basic Skills was used as a pre- and posttest. Five to 10 minutes of Brain Gym was carried out daily for one year. All of the students demonstrated a gain in reading comprehension, and 50% of the students had a gain in math skills.

Brain Gym (1998) involves activities such as cross crawls, brain buttons, and hook-ups, which are used to calm, develop better coordination between both sides of the body, draw attention to midline, reduce stress, and facilitate balance. The importance of drinking water is also stressed because the blood can carry more oxygen to the brain when it is hydrated.

Children with ASD can have difficulty with transitions. The Brain Gym exercises can signal their body to relax with clear, positive thoughts and grounding in midline during transitions (Brain Gym, 1998). Brain Gym activities are easy for parents and teachers to integrate into their routines.

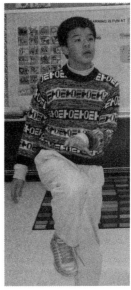

Doing Brain Gym in the classroom.

Comparison of Approaches

These five therapy approaches all involve intensive training for therapists interested in learning how to use them. Certified instructors teach in a distinct and detailed manner how to use their respective approaches with children and adults. The length of time required to become proficient varies for each approach. Each therapy method is different with regard to touch, technique, and philosophy. However, there are some similarities between the approaches.

A comparison of the complementary therapies discussed here shows that all approaches …

- ***Facilitate symmetry, balance, and a midline orientation.*** Each of these techniques is in agreement that the child's body works best from a midline orientation where both sides of the body work together in a coordinated fashion.

- *Stress the need for observation of movement of the whole body.* However, each therapy protocol uses different means to assess and facilitate a state of balanced movement. For example, NDT therapy focuses on the normal development of components of movement while emphasizing how they relate to each other and to the child as a whole in her gross-motor, fine-motor, oral-motor, and speech-language development. Craniosacral therapy (Hughes, 2004) and the Bowen Technique (Bowtech, 2006) emphasize that input to or restrictions in one part of the body affect all parts of the body. Touch for Health (1993) focuses on the triangle of health, where the emotional, nutritional, and structural aspects of the body must be in balance for health to occur. Finally, Brain Gym facilitates whole-brain learning.

- *Stress the importance of hydrating the body.* The child is encouraged to drink plenty of water before and after a Bowen session or craniosacral therapy (Hughes, 2004) to assist with removal of toxins from the body and to increase the flow of oxygenated blood to the brain and to the site of release. Drinking adequate amounts of water is also an essential part of Brain Gym (1998) and Touch for Health (1973).

- *Enhance each other in same or succeeding sessions.* After waiting the 5 to 10 days following a Bowen session, the NDT-trained therapist is better able to facilitate more normalized patterns of movement due to the child's response to the moves that reset the tension in his muscles (Bowtech, 2006). The NDT-trained therapist might also be able to facilitate these movements following a craniosacral (Hughes, 2004) treatment session, or after the body is balanced from a session using Touch for Health techniques. Finally, Brain Gym activities facilitate use of these new patterns of movement on an automatic level.

- *Require training from certified instructors.* Parents and teachers need to make sure that the therapists working with the child have received the training.

One final similarity of these complementary therapies is the need for more research. The success of all of these approaches needs to be systematically validated with children with ASD and other disorders.

Table 5.2 General Similarities Between Approaches				
NDT	Craniosacral	Bowen Technique	Touch for Health	Brain Gym

- Facilitate symmetry, a midline orientation and a balanced state
- Affect the whole body
- Stress the importance of drinking water
- Generally enhance each other when used in same or succeeding sessions
- Require training from certified instructors

Children with ASD may benefit from any of these therapies. The parent, teacher, therapist, and child must decide which would be most beneficial for the child at a particular point in time. For each of the complementary therapies, parents should seek the advice of therapists with extensive training and experience and their physicians when their child has medical complications such as intracranial pressure requiring a shunt or a seizure disorder. See the resources section in the Appendix for contact information and more details.

Case Story

The following is a case story demonstrating how the complementary therapies described in this chapter may be used in a speech-language therapy session to improve oral-motor, eating, and speech-language skills.

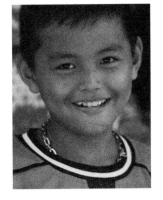

Jeremy

Jeremy is an 8-year-old boy with a diagnosis of autism. He is in the third grade at his local elementary school with a full-time aide.

Jeremy receives 60 minutes per week of speech-language therapy and 60 minutes per week of occupational therapy.

His parents contacted a private speech-language pathologist for additional therapy for disorders related to oral-motor, eating, articulation, and pragmatic language skills. The Bowen Technique (Bowtech, 2006), craniosacral therapy (Hughes, 2004), Touch for Health (1993), and the NDT approach were all incorporated into Jeremy's speech-language therapy during different therapy sessions in order to assess and facilitate his state of balance and mobility for enhanced oral-motor, eating, and speech-language skills. Although these therapies were only used in the private setting, the progress made was supported in the public school setting by using the oral-motor program presented in earlier chapters and food types that promote mature oral patterns.

Table 5.3
Jeremy's Major Difficulties

- **Poor disassociation of tongue and lip movements from jaw movements.** That is, his tongue, lips, and lower jaw all moved together during the production of oral movements, while eating, and during speech and language production.

- **Tactile defensiveness and hypersensitivity to touch around and inside his mouth.** He did not tolerate firm pressure on his face and resisted others approaching him with a Nuk brush or toothbrush.

- **Repertoire of foods was limited.** He mainly ate crunchy solids.

- **Multiple sound substitutions.** This made him difficult to understand, especially when he spoke extensively about geography or unusual animals, his special interests.

- **Poor eye contact and talking quickly without regard for his listener.** He often did not give the listener an opportunity to respond.

- **Easily overstimulated, becoming upset if the routine changed or did not happen according to his plan.** As with many children with ASD, the unfamiliar or unexpected upset him.

Treatment Program

The sessions began with Jeremy's private speech-language therapist during his individual therapy time with an evaluation of Jeremy's cranialsacral system. The speech-language therapist was trained in this technique, from which information was gained about his body symmetry, areas of restriction, his cranial rhythm, and the synchrony of movement of his cranial-sacral system. During the initial sessions, Jeremy was told what was going to happen prior to touching him. For example, the therapist said, "I'm going to touch your head now" to help reduce his tactile defensiveness. After he got used to the touch, he no longer needed to be warned each time.

The assessment of the cranialsacral system revealed restrictions at the joint of the head and the neck. Also, minimal movements were felt while monitoring his cranial rhythm at specific listening points on the body. The paired cranial bones were not moving together. After using the craniosacral techniques (Hughes, 2004), changes were observed with the synchrony of movement of the cranial bones, the amount of movement felt during monitoring of the cranial rhythm, and the amount of forward/backward movement of the head on the neck. He was then better prepared to produce mature mouth movements during the oral activities in the remainder of the session. Throughout, ongoing evaluations and treatment went hand-in-hand.

The oral-motor program followed to further prepare Jeremy for eating and speech production. It decreased his hypersensitivity to touch around and inside of the mouth and prepared his mouth for separate tongue and lip movements. The NDT approach was used to facilitate this separate movement of the tongue and lips from the lower jaw while eating. This was done through positioning for stability, support at the lower jaw, and stimulation of the side of the tongue by presenting the food at the side teeth. Jeremy then moved the food from the center of his tongue to the side, with the lower jaw and head remaining in midline. Increased lip contact was also facilitated while he chewed his food.

Next came speech production. Separate tongue movement was facilitated during the production of the /t, d, n, s/ sounds in single words selected for Jeremy through use of the PROMPT hierarchy. PROMPT, a technique developed by Deborah Hayden (Chumpelik, 1984), stands for "Prompts for Restructuring Oral Muscular Phonetic Targets." Production of the targeted speech sounds was assisted through use of the PROMPT techniques during a structured language activity. It was easier for Jeremy to produce these speech sounds following the oral-motor program because it decreased his hypersensitivity to touch inside of his mouth.

The changes that occurred during this therapy session included increased mobility, balance and organization of the body, decreased oral hypersensitivity, increased stability of the body, and separate movement of the tongue and lips while eating and speaking. These changes were a result of (a) craniosacral therapy (Hughes, 2004); (b) the oral-motor program, which helped to facilitate normal movement patterns; (c) the NDT approach; and (d) the PROMPT technique (Chumpelik, 1984). Jeremy's whole body was treated during this speech-language therapy session, resulting in mature oral movements while eating and speaking.

The next session began with a Touch for Health (1973) balance. A 14-muscle check was performed to assess areas of muscle imbalance. The balancing procedures determined whether the right and left sides and the front and back of the body were working together. The muscle check also provided information about areas to work on with Jeremy during the third session when the Bowen Technique was used.

Following the third session, a decision was made to continue using the Bowen Technique. At this point in time, Jeremy responded best to specific moves with wait time off the body at the end of each series of moves.

The oral-motor program and production of the targeted speech sounds through use of the PROMPT technique (Chumpelik, 1984) followed the Bowen Technique. The goal of this session, and all the sessions, was always to improve Jeremy's oral-motor function during eating and speech-language production. The Bowen Technique, the oral-motor program, and the PROMPT technique were used to meet this goal.

Summary

The complementary therapies discussed here can be used together or individually. Mari Miyoshi, occupational therapist, in "OT Teams with Other Modalities to Boost Whole Brain Learning," stated that craniosacral therapy and Brain Gym can be used together to help children develop "whole brain learning" (Miyoshi, 2004, p. 48).

The NDT approach (NDT), craniosacral therapy, the Bowen Technique, Touch for Health, and Brain Gym can each be used to facilitate balanced, symmetrical movements for improved oral-motor, eating, and speech-language skills. With these techniques and the oral-motor program as part of the overall speech-language treatment strategy, the child can make changes that become systematically joined into his whole body on an automatic level. Ultimately, because the child's body is now in a more balanced state, he can approach his optimal level of functioning while eating, during speech-language production, as well as during spontaneous verbal and nonverbal communication. The child can adapt to sensory information presented to him and make use of it to develop sensory-motor maps, and plan and produce movements. Ideally, these sensory-motor maps will be available for the child to repeat in other situations. ■

CHAPTER 6

Summary and Conclusions

The goal of this book is to help parents and teachers understand why it is important to evaluate and treat the oral-motor skills of the child who has a diagnosis of autism spectrum disorders (ASD) and how to incorporate work on oral-motor skills into routines over the course of the day. Often therapists recommend that parents and teachers do certain activities with the child without telling them why they are important. This book gives the "why" and "how." When the importance of working on specific skills is explained, parents and teachers become more invested in the treatment, more consistent in performing the treatment, and more creative in finding ways to work on the child's skills in their daily routines. As long as you understand why a particular goal is important for the child, you can work on it in almost any situation with most materials, such as a regular toothbrush, a lollipop, a wet washcloth, or some lotion. Parents and teachers can then become active participants in the child's treatment program, which is also a goal of this book.

Through case studies and references to existing research, this book has shown how improved oral-motor skills facilitate the development of eating skills, speech production, and eventually communication skills. Most important, this simple treatment program can be easily incorporated into the child's daily schedule for maximum effectiveness. ■

References

Alexander, R., Boehme, R., & Cupps, B. (1982). *Early feeding, sound production, and pre-linguistic/cognitive development and their relationship to gross-motor and fine-motor development* [Handout]. Wauwatosa, WI.

American Psychiatric Association. (2000). *Diagnostic and statistical manual of mental disorders* (4th ed.; text revision). Washington, DC: Author.

Anderson, T. (2001). *Different types of exercise.* Retrieved September 9, 2006, from www.trulyhuge.com/news/tips55a.htm

Apraxia-Kids. (2005). *Understanding apraxia.* Retrieved December 2, 2005, from www.apraxiakids.org/site/apps/nl/content3.asp?c=chKMIOPIIsE7b=787891&ct=46

Augustyniak, R. (2005). The art of bowen. Bowen hands. *The Journal of Bowen Therapy Academy of Australia, 14*(1), 8-10.

Ayres, J. A. (1979). *Sensory integration and the child.* Los Angeles: Western Psychological Services.

Beckman, D. (1995a*).* Major brain centers for oral motor control. *Oral Motor Assessment & Intervention,* 11-12.

Beckman, D. (1995b). Oral-motor patterns. *Oral Motor Assessment & Intervention,* 20-31.

Bobath, B., & Bobath, K. (1975). *Motor development in different types of cerebral palsy.* London: The Whitefriars Ltd.

Bowtech. (2006). *How it works.* Retrieved March 3, 2007, from www.bowtech.com

Brain Gym. (1998). Retrieved March 3, 2007, from www.braingym.org

Chumpelik, D. (1984). The PROMPT system of therapy: Theoretical framework and applications for developmental apraxia of speech. *Seminars in Speech and Language, 5,* 139-156.

Clark, H. M. (2006). *Therapeutic exercise in dysphagia management: Philosophies, practices, and challenges.* American Speech-Language-Hearing Association (ASHA). Professional Development & Special Interest Division 13, Swallowing and Swallowing Disorders (Dysphagia).

Evans-Morris, S., & Dunn-Klein, M. (1987). *Pre-feeding skills.* Tucson, AZ: Therapy Skill Builders.

Escalona, A., Field, T., & Singer-Strunch, R., Cullen, C., Hartshorn, K. (2001). Improvements in the behavior of children with autism following massage therapy. *Journal of Autism Dev. Disorders, 31*(5), 513-516.

Field, T. (2001). *The importance of touch.* Retrieved July 15, 2006, from http://www.karger.com/gazette/67/Field/art_4.htm

Gagnon, D. E. (2003). *Tone versus strength.* Retrieved January 20, 2008, from www.dsnetworkaz.mykb.com/Article_28418.aspx

Genna, C. W. (2001). Tactile defensiveness and other sensory modulation difficulties. *LEAVEN, 37*(3), 51-53.

Government Reform Committee of the U.S. House of Representatives, 106th Congress. (1999-2000). *Autism-observations, experiences and concepts.* Washington, DC: Upledger, John D.O.

Gustafson, S. (2007). *Maternal & newborn care.* Retrieved August 21, 2007, from www.bowtech.com/articles/maternal-newborn-care_2html

Hannaford, C. (1995). *Smart moves. Why learning is not all in your head.* Arlington, VA: Great Ocean Publishers.

Henry, S., & Myles, B. S. (2007). *The comprehensive autism planning system (CAPS) for individuals with Asperger Syndrome, autism and related disabilities: Integrating best practices throughout the student's day.* Shawnee Mission, KS: Autism Asperger Publishing Company.

Hoekman, L. A. (2005). *Sensory integration.* Retrieved August 13, 2005, from, http://www.thegraycenter.org

Howle, J. (2002). *Neuro-developmental treatment approach: Theoretical foundations and principles of clinical practice.* Laguna Beach, CA: Neuro-Developmental Treatment Association.

Hughes, D. (2004). *An interview with Dr. John Upledger.* Retrieved July 25, 2007, from www.shareguide.com/Upledger.html

King, L. J. (1991). Sensory integration: An effective approach to therapy and education. *Autism Research Review International, 5*, 2.

King, L. J. (2002a). *Tactile system.* Retrieved October 15, 2005, from http://www.thechildrenscenteraz.org/tactile.htm

King, L. J. (2002b). *Understanding proprioception.* Retrieved October 15, 2005, from http://www.thechildrenscenteraz.org/proprioceptive.htm

King, L. J. (2002c). *Vestibular system.* Retrieved October 15, 2005, from http://www.thechildrenscenteraz.org/vestibular.htm

Kumin, L. (2002). Developmental apraxia of speech in children and adults with down syndrome. *Disability Solutions, 5*, 1-15.

Lawrence, M. (1971). Mechanics of the ear. In L. E. Travis (Ed.), *Handbook of speech pathology and audiology* (pp. 245-261). New York: Appleton-Century-Crofts Educational Division Meredith Corporation.

Lazarus, C. L. (2006). *Lingual strengthening and swallowing.* Rockville, MD: American Speech-Language-Hearing Association (ASHA). Professional Development & Special Interest Division 13, Swallowing and Swallowing Disorders (Dysphagia).

Logemann, J. A. (2006). *Medical and rehabilitative therapy of oral, pharyngeal motor disorders.* Retrieved September 9, 2006, from http://www.nature.com/gimo/contents/pt1/full/gimo50.html

Lucker-Lazerson, N. (2003). *Apraxia? Dyspraxia? Articulation? Phonology? What does it all mean.* Retrieved December 2, 2005, from www.apraxia-kids.org/site/apps/nl/content3.asp?c=ch

Manipulative and body-based practices: an overview. (2007). Backgrounder. Retrieved December 2, 2007, from www.nccam.nih.gov/health/backgrounds/manipulative.htm

Marshalla, P. (2001). *Becoming verbal with childhood apraxia.* Kirkland, WI: Marshalla Speech and Language.

Mayer-Johnson (1994-2005). *The Picture Communication Symbols Libraries, Boardmaker, Writing with Symbols.* Solana Beach, CA: Mayer-Johnson, LLC.

Miyoshi, M. (2004, March). OT teams with other modalities to boost whole brain learning. *Your Health Magazine*, 48.

Moller, A. R. (2006). *Hearing: anatomy, physiology and disorders of the auditory system.* Burlington, MA: Academic Press.

Murdoch, B. E., Ozanne, A. E., & Cross, J. A. (1990). Acquired childhood speech/disorders: dysarthria and dyspraxia. In R. Bonnett, B. E. Murdoch, & M. E. Murdoch (Eds.), *Acquired neurological speech/language disorders in childhood* (pp. 308-341). London: Taylor and Francis.

Myles, B. S., Cook, K. T., Miller, N. E., Rinner, L., & Robbins, L. A. (2000). *Asperger Syndrome and sensory issues: Practical solutions for making sense of the world.* Shawnee Mission, KS: Autism Asperger Publishing Company.

Neuro-Developmental Treatment Association (NDT). *Welcome to NDT.* Retrieved August 22, 2007, from www.ndta.org

Rapin, I. (1997). Autism. *The New England Journal of Medicine, 337*(2), 97-104.

Redstone, F. (2004). The importance of postural control for feeding (in children with neurogenic disorders). *Pediatric Nursing, 30*(2), 97-100.

Redstone, F. (2007). Neurodevelopmental treatment in speech-language pathology: theory, practice, and research. *Communicative Disorders Review, 1*(2), 119-131.

Rehabilitation Institute of Chicago. Communicative Disorders Care Committee. (2002). *What is dysarthria?* Retrieved December 2, 2005, from http://lifecenter.ric.org/content/280/?topic=1&subtopic=300

Richardson, G. (2004). Sam- a heart wrenching story. Bowen Hands. *The Journal of Bowen Therapy Academy of Australia, 13*(3), 3-5.

Sheppard, J. J. (2006). *The role of oral sensorimotor therapy in the treatment of pediatric dysphagia.* Rockville, MD: American Speech-Language-Hearing Association (ASHA). Professional Development & Special Interest Division 13, Swallowing and Swallowing Disorders (Dysphagia).

Touch for Health. (1973). *Techniques.* Retrieved March 3, 2007, from www.touchfor-health.com

Upledger, J. (2001). Craniosacral therapy and attention deficit disorder. *Massage Today, 01*, 8. Retrieved July 25, 2007, from www.massagetoday.com/mpacms/mt/article.php?id=10305

Whitaker, J. A., Gilliam, P. P., & Seba, D. B. (1997). *The Bowen Technique: A gentle hands-on method that affects the autonomic nervous system as measured by heart rate variability and clinical assessment.* Retrieved July 21, 2007, from www.bowtech.com/bowen-research/completed-research.html

Yack, E., Aquilla, P., & Sutton, S. (2002). *Building bridges through sensory integration. Therapy for children with autism and other pervasive developmental disorders.* Arlington, TX: Future Horizons.

Yost, W. A. (2002). Auditory perception. In *The encyclopedia of the human brain* (Volume 1, A-Cog, pp. 303-320). New York: Academic Press.

Appendix

Oral-Motor/Eating/Speech Checklist

Name: _____

Birthdate: _____

Age: _____

Date: _____

I. Oral Structures/Musculature During Movement
I: (imitation)   S: (spontaneous)

(*Note: asymmetries, movement patterns, and ability to produce separate movements*)

1. Open mouth: _____

2. Close mouth: _____

3. Smile: _____

4. Pucker: _____

5. Blow: _____

6. Hum: _____

7. Oo-ee:_____

8. Lip smack: _____

9. Puff out cheeks: _____

10. Tongue out (with mouth open): _____

11. Tongue out/in (with mouth open): _____

12. Tongue tip up inside of mouth: _____

13. Tongue tip to upper lip: _____

14. Tongue tip down inside of mouth: _____

15. Tongue tip to lower lip: _____

Flanagan, M. (2008). *Improving speech and eating skills in children with autism spectrum disorders: An oral-motor program for home and school.* Shawnee Mission, KS: Autism Asperger Publishing Company. www.asperger.net. Used with permission.

16. Tongue side to side to mouth corners: _____

17. Tongue side to side to lower teeth: _____

18. Tongue side to side to cheeks: _____

19. Tongue side to side to upper teeth: _____

20. Tongue click: _____

21. Click teeth: _____

II. *Oral and Postural Muscle Tone*

1. Facial tone: _____

2. Lingual tone: _____

3. Body tone: _____

III. *Respiration*

1. Oral breather: _____

2. Nasal breather: _____

IV. *Movements While Eating*

1. Food texture prefer: _____

2. Food texture avoid: _____

3. Description of movements with:

    A. liquid: _____

        a. cup: _____

        b. straw: _____

    B. semi-solid from a spoon: _____

    C. soft solid: _____

    D. hard solid: _____

Flanagan, M. (2008). *Improving speech and eating skills in children with autism spectrum disorders: An oral-motor program for home and school.* Shawnee Mission, KS: Autism Asperger Publishing Company. www.asperger.net. Used with permission.

V. *Vocal Quality*

1. Normal: _____

2. Breathy: _____

3. Harsh: _____

4. Hoarse: _____

5. Nasal: _____

6. De-nasal: _____

7. High pitch: _____

8. Low or high volume level: _____

VI. *Speech-Language Production*

1. Sound play: _____

2. Gestures/sign language: _____

3. Sound imitation: _____

4. Word imitation: _____

Flanagan, M. (2008). *Improving speech and eating skills in children with autism spectrum disorders: An oral-motor program for home and school.* Shawnee Mission, KS: Autism Asperger Publishing Company. www.asperger.net. Used with permission.

Materials for Oral-Motor Box/Bag

1. A variety of brushes:

    -   Nuk massage brush – oval-shaped brush designed for infants to help them become accustomed to teeth-brushing. It is frequently used by therapists for oral stimulation with children to stimulate the tongue, palate, inside of the cheeks, lips, and gums. It is important not to use this for biting or chewing.

    -   proPreefer – another type of brush for the tongue – not a chew toy

    -   battery-operated toothbrush

    -   toothbrush – The toothbrush should be small and soft.

    -   Toothettes/dental swabs

    -   finger brushes

2. Mini massagers
    These may be of a variety of sizes and speeds. If the massager is too fast for the child, the battery may be run out until it is at an acceptable speed.

3. Flavored tongue depressors

4. Chewy tubes: The chewy tube can be in the shape of a T, P, or Q so that the child or therapist/parent can hold on to one end while the child chews on the other end.

5. Flavored gloves – gloves that taste like cherry, grape, etc.

6. Flavor sprays – sprays of different flavors

7. A variety of whistles/hum-a-zoos – a toy the child hums into.

8. Bubbles: Regular or candy bubbles

9. Lollipops: Especially the small, round lollipops

10. ChapSticks: These may be purchased in a variety of flavors, giving the child an opportunity to communicate a choice

11. Washcloths: the small, baby washcloths work best

12. Lotion

13. Powder

14. Powder puffs

15. Hand mitts

16. Oral-motor exercise playing cards

Oral-Motor Program Data Sheet

NAME:

	Date (A) accept (R) reject	Date (A) accept (R) reject	Date (A) accept (R) reject
1. Lotion			
a. body:			
b. face:			
2. ChapStick			
3. Nuk brush			
a. lips:			
b. tongue:			
inside of mouth:			
outside of mouth:			
sides of the tongue:			
4. Chew tube			
a. consecutive chew:			
b. right side:			
c. left side:			
5. Other			

Flanagan, M. (2008). *Improving speech and eating skills in children with autism spectrum disorders: An oral-motor program for home and school.* Shawnee Mission, KS: Autism Asperger Publishing Company. www.asperger.net. Used with permission.

Glossary

Abnormal development: This refers to skills or behaviors that would not be seen with the child's typical peers.

Apraxia: A motor speech disorder where there is difficulty planning the movements and sequences of sounds for speech production.

Auditory system: The sense of hearing through which we receive and process information.

Autism spectrum disorder (ASD): A developmental disorder that is characterized by deficits in social interactions, language, communication and play, with stereotypic, repetitive behaviors and a narrow range of interests.

Autonomic nervous system (ANS): Part of the peripheral nervous system that controls such functions as heart rate, respiration rate, digestion and perspiration.

Aversion: A desire to avoid something or someone.

Babble: A normal stage in speech-language development that occurs between 6 and 7 months. The child produces long, rhythmical sequences of the same consonant and vowel sounds.

Cheek/lip retraction: Pulling back of the cheeks and lips due to increased muscle tone restricting movement.

Chew tube: A solid, washable, non-toxic tube used to facilitate chewing and biting skills.

Delayed development: Development of the same skills as typical peers but at a slower rate.

Distal: Relating to being away from the middle or center of the body.

Dysarthria: A motor speech disorder that involves difficulty with speech due to incoordination or weakness of the musculature.

Fight or flight: A hyper-alert state used for survival.

Gag reflex: A protective oral reflex in response to harmful or unknown stimuli.

Hypertonia: High or increased muscle tone.

Hypotonia: Low or decreased muscle tone.

Hypersensitivity: Over-reactive to sensation.

Hypo-sensitivity: Under-reactive to sensation.

Imitation: Mimicking or copying gross-, fine-, or speech movements.

Inhibition: To prevent or stop from overreacting or occurring.

Initiate: To take the first turn.

Isometric exercise: An exercise used to train the strength of a muscle or muscle group.

Jargoning: A stage in normal development where there is a variety of sounds sequenced with varied inflection.

Jaw clenching: Tightly closing the jaw in a clamped position.

Joint attention: A shared attention of an object or event with another person.

Muscle tone: State of tension or readiness of a muscle to respond to a stretch.

Mobility: Capable of moving.

Modulate: The facilitation of some neural messages while inhibiting other neural messages when producing a response.

Motor planning: The ability to cognitively organize and produce a sequence of novel movements.

Nuk massage brush: An oval-shaped brush produced for infants to assist with their ability to become accustomed to teeth-brushing. It is frequently used by therapists to provide oral stimulation.

Oral apraxia: A disorder involving difficulty with the production of volitional oral movements such as sticking out your tongue or licking your lips, even when the child is capable of producing these movements.

Oral-motor: The ability to purposefully move the lips, tongue, cheeks, palate, and jaw with stability, grading, and separation due to an intact sensory-motor feedback system.

Oral structures: The lips, cheeks, tongue, teeth, jaw, gums, and palate.

Primitive movements: Movements seen in the infant during the first three to four months of development (e.g., oral reflexes).

Proprioceptive system: The sensory system that gives us information from the sensory receptors in our muscles and joints. This system gives information about what the body is doing in space.

Proximal: Located toward the center of the body.

Register: To notice and pay attention to.

Sensory input: The information that goes from the sensory receptors to the brain.

Sensory integration: The ability to organize and use sensory information to interact with the environment.

Signs: Hand and finger movements that have meaning and are used for communication.

Stability: Being steady and balanced.

Tactile defensiveness: A condition due to difficulty modulating sensory input, which causes the child to react negatively to touch.

Tactile system: The system where sensory input is received by the sensory receptors in the skin and sent to the central nervous system.

Tongue retraction: A pulling back of the tongue into the mouth. The tip of the tongue may be held up against the palate.

Tongue thrust: A forceful forward movement of the tongue.

Vestibular system: This sensory system, located in the inner ear, registers changes in gravity and influences muscle tone, movement and balance.

Resources

Organizations

American Speech/Language Hearing Assn.
10801 Rockville Pike
Rockville, MD 20852
(800) 638-8255
www.asha.org

Brain Gym International
1575 Spinaker Drive
Suite 204 B
Ventura, CA   93001
800-356-2109
www.braingym.com

Neuro-Developmental Treatment Assn.
1540 S. Coast Highway, Ste. 203
Laguna Beach, CA 92651
800-869-9295
www.ndta.org

Touch for Health Education
Matthew Thie
6162 La Gloria Drive
Malibu, CA 90265
310-589-5269
www.touch4health.com

United States Bowen Registry
337 North Rush Street
Prescott, AZ 86301
1-928-772-2493
www.bowtech.com

Upledger Institute
11211 Prosperity Farms Road, Suite D-223
Palm Beach Gardens, FL 33410
1-561-622-4334
www.upledger.com

Companies That Sell Oral-Motor Products

Mayer-Johnson LLC
P. O. Box 1579
Solana Beach, CA 92075-7579
800-588-4548
www.mayer-johnson.com

Pocket Full of Therapy
P.O. Box 174
Morganville, NJ 07751
732-441-1422
www.pfot.com

Southpaw Enterprises
P. O. Box 1047
Dayton, OH 45401-1047
800-228-1698
www.southpawenterprises.com

Super Duper Publications
Dept. SD 2008, P. O. Box 24997
Greenville, SC 29616-2497
800-277-8737
www.superduperinc.com

The Speech Bin
P. O. Box 922668
Norcross, GA 30010-2668
800-850-8602
www.speechbin.com

Therapy Shoppe, Inc.
P. O. Box 8875
Grand Rapids, MI 49518
800-261-5590
www.therapyshoppe.com

APC

Autism Asperger Publishing Company
P.O. Box 23173
Shawnee Mission, Kansas 66283-0173
877-277-8254
www.asperger.net